The Broken Heart
Protect Your Heart from Daily Stress and Emotional Upheavals

by

Tali T. Bashour M.D.FACC

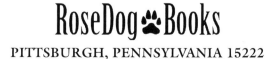

RoseDog✿Books

PITTSBURGH, PENNSYLVANIA 15222

RoseDog Books
701 Smithfield Street
Pittsburgh, PA 15222
Visit our website at www.rosedogbookstore.com

ISBN: 978-1-4349-8399-2
eISBN: 978-1-4349-4648-5

ENDORSEMENT BY LEADERS IN THE FIELD

DEDICATIONS

To my wife Mary Anne, for being my right hand all along. By the way I am right-handed! Also to Karen, Keenan, and Ryan my very loving and supportive children

CONTENTS

ACKNOWLEDGEMENTS

The Author acknowledges the valuable advice from all who volunteered to help in this project. They include many physicians, nurses, other health care professionals, as well as other individuals from the public at large. To all, I cannot thank you enough.

"Yes My Friend, I Believe"

On a day in February 1994, my phone rang and it was an old friend and colleague whom I had not seen in months. He was objecting to a press release I gave to a local San Mateo Newspaper. He was referring to a recent medical study I presented in Budapest. I then warned that emotionally "Broken Hearts" can suffer true heart attacks.

"Do you really believe that? He asked, and I replied: "You know I am a clinical researcher and a physician. I do believe in my objective findings. I have done three different studies that all show a link between emotional stress and heart damage." I then recited several case histories. My friend remained unconvinced but puzzled and clearly fascinated. Nearly a decade later, scholars in Japan, the United States and Europe all started publishing papers about the heart as a victim of stress hormones unleashed either by emotional shock, or sustained emotional stress.

The hormones constrict the coronary arteries that supply the heart with oxygen and nutrition leading to breakdown of heart muscle tissue.

Medical Histories in this book represent real patients whose names were withheld or changed.

EMILY'S HEART

Emily had a good heart; literally and metaphorically. Her heart was healthy, with good arteries and strong muscle. It responded perfectly to its own electrical stimulation and passed all tests given by her doctor. Emily also had a loving heart. Her husband had passed away ten years earlier, but she was close to her grandchildren, a boy and a girl - especially the girl, Lilly. Emily loved Lilly dearly. She played with her almost every day and even started teaching her French, the language of her own parents. And then, suddenly, Lilly died of acute leukemia.

Emily felt a tight band compressing her chest, and found it hard to breathe. She didn't know her heart was pumping at only a quarter of its normal power. Medications were prescribed to help strengthen Emily's heart and ease the pressure, but the medicine could not remove the image of Lilly.

As Emily's cardiologist I admitted her to the hospital and sat with her the next morning to explain that she was suffering from a newly recognized problem: broken heart syndrome.

"Chances are you will recover in about a week," I told her. Family, friends, and the nursing staff were all supportive. When she worried and wondered if she would ever really recover, I told her about many similar patients whom I treated for this condition.

*Brian, a 35 year-old man suffered from chest pain a few minutes after a heavy metal bar fell upon his head. As the chest pain worsened it became harder for him to breathe and he was rushed to the Emergency Room (ER).

*Sarah, a 75 year old woman who had a long stand history of high blood pressure, developed brain hemorrhage. She became breathless and had severe congestion in her lungs.

*Mark, a 30 year-old man, was vacationing in Japan when a major earthquake occurred. The shock of the huge quake startled Mark into sudden chest pain and wheezing. His lungs filled up with fluid and he was rushed to the nearest ER.

*29 year-old Jenny was addicted to methamphetamines. One day, she took more speed than usual. A terrible pain in her chest sent her to the ER.

*At the age of 64, Wilma's heart seemed to be weakening. The doctors discovered a tumor on her adrenal gland. They found it to be "benign," but secreting excessive amounts of adrenaline.

*James had been preparing his speech for weeks, practicing in front of his wife and the mirror. On the big day, he was extremely stressed out and collapsed while giving the speech.

*For 75-year-old Robert, the loss of his grandson in a car accident was devastating. He developed chest pain and was taken to the nearest ER.

All these people suffered from broken heart syndrome: a traumatic emotional experience that causes powerful emotions to weaken the heart. Within two weeks, all of them had recovered.

Broken heart syndrome occurs when a sudden shock or repeated stress stimulates the adrenal gland or the sympathetic nerve centers in the brain. The body then produces stress hormones, such as adrenalin, that gush into the bloodstream and flood the heart. The pressure of these hormones constricts the coronary arteries that supply the heart with oxygen and nutrition, and the heart muscles break down.

This book highlights the complex connection between emotions and the body, and how the stresses of daily life, work, family problems, unmet financial needs, conflicts, wars, and natural disasters take a heavy toll on our hearts. It doesn't have to. When people learn to deal with these situations through exercise and diet management they will discover the key to a healthy heart.

Emotional situations exert their harmful effects on the human heart through a joint pathway or mechanism. By "whipping" the adrenal gland[*1] (located on tops of the kidneys) or by stimulating the sympa-

---

* located at the top of each kidney adrenal glands secrete stress and hormones such as adrenaline and noradrenaline intended to rally the support system to defend the body at time of crisis.

thetic nerve centers in the brain, they can rapidly flood the blood stream with stress hormones. These hormones, such as adrenaline, are known as catecholamines. They are meant to rally body defenses to cope with a shocking situation or a looming disaster; however, they may create an overkill that devastates the heart muscle. A condition recently described as the "Broken Heart" is caused by powerful stimulation that catches the heart so off guard and unprepared that it may be forced to give in. Quite often the Broken Heart condition is brought about by a heightened emotional reaction to a sudden dilemma.

INTRODUCTION
EMOTIONAL HEART DISEASE
THE BROKEN HEART: FICTION, SCIENCE, OR PLAIN POETRY?

Throughout civilizations, the landscapes of emotions and the human heart have been contested, being jointly or alternately claimed, disclaimed, and reclaimed by scientists, novelists, artists and poets alike. The heart is, after all, the first organ to react to powerful emotions. This includes feelings of palpitation* due to either rapid or powerful heartbeats or both. Other manifestations include heaviness in the heart area or in the throat. To add to the confusion, the symptom of "blacking out" or fainting, medically termed "syncope," can result from sudden emotional stimulation as well as from actual heart disease. Past cultures considered the heart to be the center of emotions such as love, hate, and sadness in particular. Today, the heart is not viewed as the instigator of emotions, but merely as their interpreter, and occasionally their victim.

From where then does the source of emotional flow originate? Today's scientists agree that these feelings flow directly from the brain, or varying sites within. Basic emotions - including joy, sadness, fear, disgust, and surprise - stem from certain locations in the brain, while love, hate, jealousy and other more complex and less understood feel-

---

*palpitation: powerful or rapid heart beat

ings may represent a combination of basic emotions, frequently handled by higher brain centers.

So, do we know for sure that our emotional outpouring flows from the brain? Scientists seek proof. Aided by amazing new technologies such as Functional Magnetic Resonance Imaging (FMRI), they are able to probe certain areas of the brain and even indentify processes such as falling in love, fearing a real (or imaginary) adversity, and not being truthful. Zones in active functional phases "light up" and become brighter indicating increased activity. With more refined scanners and sophisticated software, it is likely that scientists will have the ability to read one's mind and even digitally reconstruct images of his thoughts. This will all contribute to our understanding of how our hearts and heads are linked.

If the heart is indeed a victim and a theatre on which emotions play profound influence, how can an emotional release adversely affect and disrupt heart function? First let us examine the normal heart function. The heart is predominantly a mechanical pump. In order to perform properly and distribute nutrition to all organs, it needs to be nourished as well. This sustenance is provided by the coronary arteries, originating in the aorta and descending into the heart muscle. Any severe narrowing or complete blockage in one or more of these arteries can result in varying degrees of abnormalities in heart performance, ranging from suboptimal function to actual damage that can cause permanent loss of function of the affected area. Traditionally, this has been attributed to a common condition called "atherosclerosis," a process that leads to clogging of arteries by cholesterol, blood components and inflammatory cellular reactions. Certain predisposing factors are now unequivocally proven and they include high blood pressure, diabetes, abnormal cholesterol and lipid patterns, tobacco smoking, and other genetically transmitted traits.

The other mechanism of heart injury is heart muscle exhaustion as a consequence of overstimulation, or overloading from leaky valves, or from increased flow resistance commonly due to high blood pressure. A host of other agents can directly weaken the heart including certain viral infections, toxic chemicals, and abuse of alcohol, or certain other drugs.

Through the known history of human intellect, emotional stress has been suspected to play a major role in the condition of the heart. It is now accepted that potent emotions can, by stimulating the release of stress hormones such as catecholamines (adrenaline is the main one), affect the arteries - by dynamically constricting them (spasm) - and the heart muscle-by causing further weakening. In an extreme case the heart may become stunned and lose much of its pumping function (The Broken Heart). Fortunately, the process is reversible in most cases, over the course of days, with subsequent recovery of much, if not all, of heart muscle function.

Legends of love and hate, historic happenings, poetic metaphors and colorful artistic expressions all illustrate the earliest suspicions of the relationship between our emotions and our hearts. I will attempt throughout the pages of this book to illuminate this relationship through stories, historical and literary, and those of my own medical experience. The images of these characters will amplify the concepts of how emotional surges can disrupt the integrity and the harmony of the working heart, occasionally endangering its very function of maintaining life.

While many heart conditions are not directly linked to emotions; most are profoundly influenced by emotional instability. One can also wonder whether all emotional activities are bad for the heart. The correct answer is, "probably not." Emotions are a natural part of our human experience and a reasonable "dose" of emotions can be potentially beneficial. Just like physical exercise, emotional activity stimulates the heart, increases pulse rate, and can, therefore, enhance the training and endurance of the heart as an organ. Emotional fitness, as much as physical fitness, is essential for good health.

Manifestations of emotional heart disease that will be discussed in detail include:

(1.) Chest pain (angina) in middle-aged women within the period that extends from shortly before menopause to several years after.

(2.) Heart attacks or sudden deaths occurring shortly after learning of a major tragedy, such as the loss of a beloved person.

(3.) Heart attacks after acute and profound emotional stress without previously known heart disease.

(4.) Fainting (syncope) at major and profoundly disturbing news, or upon facing a sudden perplexing situation.

(5.) Acute and severe worsening of heart function without a heart attack, especially after the unexpected loss of loved ones - a condition often referred to as "stunned heart".

(6.) Sustained stress as a risk factor for heart attacks and premature death.

To what degree should we interfere to protect the heart from suffering emotional havoc is yet another medically complex and potentially disturbing issue, both anthropologically and ethically. Should we manipulate our emotions to escape their potentially damaging effects? Or should we focus on how to protect our hearts from absolute emotional tyranny?

Please recognize the novelty of this subject. Being at a stage of scientific infancy, new revelations are expected to emerge as socio-medical research continues to unlock the secrets of the historic link between emotions and the human heart.

Let us start our journey together and learn first what can go wrong with the heart in general, and where emotional heart disease fits in this large scheme. The two "landscapes" most affected by emotional stress are, first, the coronary arteries on which the heart is totally dependent for its nutrition and therefore survival, and second, the heart muscle itself. Let us learn more about these two targeted systems.

CHAPTER ONE

CORONARY HEART DISEASE

"Number one on the "Most Wanted List"

CORONARY HEART DISEASE

The term Coronary Heart Disease (CHD) reflects a compromised heart function due to reduced blood flow through the coronary arteries that carry nutrition to the heart muscle, also known as the myocardium. This muscle, when stimulated by a special electrical system, contracts and pumps out the blood from heart chambers. CHD is the number one cause of death and incapacitation in the United States and much of the western world, with rapidly rising incidence in the developing nations as well. This disease assaults its victims in different ways. Sometimes it can cause rapid death by sudden electrical chaos which renders the heart muscle function totally impotent. And sometimes it can bring about systematic massive "destruction" of functioning heart muscle, as in acute myocardial infarction (heart attack), which often results in life-threatening heart failure. The killing process can yet take a third form of slowly progressive damage of the heart muscle, eventually leading to ongoing and disabling heart failure which is, nowadays, one of the most frequent incapacitating chronic medical conditions in this country. On a hopeful note and thanks to successive medical breakthroughs, this rampant plague appears to be losing some of its seemingly unchallengeable power. Death related to coronary heart disease is finally declining in the United States.

Youth and Gender did *NOT* Protect Her.

When she was seen in my office on referral by her family physician, Vera Santos had celebrated her 37th birthday two days earlier.

3

However, she had not been feeling well for over three weeks. She described having chest "pressure" merging with an aching sensation in the middle of her chest. This feeling spread to her neck area and left arm whenever she walked fast or climbed stairs. She was predictably relieved after sitting or resting for five minutes. With such a complaint, practically ever physician would consider a condition called "**Angina Pectoris**" or Chest Pain due to lack of adequate blood supply to the heart. At her young age she had already been diagnosed with diabetes, high cholesterol and high blood pressure. Her immediate family had more than their fair share of coronary heart disease, her 32-year-old brother and 42-year-old sister had both died from heart attacks in the Philippines. An older brother living in the USA had a stent implanted in his coronary artery to treat chest pain. And even though her father was never diagnosed with heart disease, he died from a massive stroke.

My diagnosis was coronary artery disease. However, it is mandatory to confirm this with further testing. The simplest approach would be to do a **Treadmill Stress Echo Test.*** Her test was strongly abnormal. Severe disease was found in two coronary arteries out of the three major ones. I advised Vera to have stents placed in the two diseased arteries. The procedure was successful. Her only regret was that her siblings in her native country were never given the chance she had.

Over the centuries, the concept of a weakened heart has fueled both intensive scientific research as well as passionate poetic verses. It is only in the modern era of science that indisputable identifiable underlying causes - referred to as risk factors - have been firmly established as the real culprits. Among several predisposing causes, five stand out as both most common and most serious. These include:

1) Hypertension (high blood pressure), 2) diabetes, 3) elevated blood levels of harmful fats such as cholesterol and triglycerides or a low level of the "good cholesterol" known as High Density Lipoprotein (HDL), 4) smoking nicotine cigarettes, 5) genetic factors, and 6) emotional stress.

Any of these factors, alone or especially in combinations of two or more, can lead to the disease scientifically called atherosclerosis, a.k.a "hardening of the arteries." This condition is characterized by infiltration of lipids (fat substances) and a host of cells and chemical factors under the lining of arteries, eventually leading to constricted size of the opening (lumen), and subsequent reduction in blood flow. What hap-

---

* Stress Echo Test is an exercise test with echocardiographic recording which makes it quite sensitive for diagnosing CHD

pens next is a reduction of delivery of oxygen and nutritional materials to the working body organs including the heart, brain, legs, kidneys, and many others, none of which can escape the harmful effects of this "starvation."

"A Starved Heart": What are the Signs?

Let us continue and try to understand how hardened arteries can have damaging effects on the heart and how this damage manifests. Chest pain, known as "angina pectoris," is often the first symptom commonly described by patients as a compressing, painful sensation in the front of the chest, occurring typically after physical activity and relieved by resting. Unfortunately, the onset of this symptom is late and usually after the disease in the arteries has already progressed to an advanced stage. Often a multiplicity of medications or intervention will be needed, including coronary bypass operations or angioplasty, the less invasive mechanical-expansion of narrowed arteries using balloons or stents.*

Unfortunately, the condition can be either silent or associated only with mild discomfort commonly not raising major concerns. Many patients often attribute the feeling to "stomach upset" or "heart burn". The lack of pain is commonly observed in diabetic patients in particular, who may even suffer unrecognized "silent" heart attacks leading to a serious compromise in heart function and eventually heart failure.

As a rule angina occurs when an artery is significantly narrowed but not totally occluded. Failure to increase the blood flow in such an artery as a response to increased demand during physical activity will lead to chest pain. On the other hand, a heart attack is usually the consequence of sudden total blockage of the artery, frequently by a blood clot. Let's assume that this same person with severe coronary artery disease is subjected to an emotional reaction or acute anxiety. It is likely that his heart may not be able to tolerate the added load, leading to an aggravation of symptoms and probably even more serious consequences.

---

* Stents are cylindrical nets made of metals that can be implanted via arteries in a nonsurgical technique and expand to dilate the constricted segments of the coronary arteries. The procedure is commonly referred to as "Angioplasty". Initially introduced by Dr. Andreas Gruntzig from Switzerland using balloons delivered by arterial catheters to dilate the narrowed coronary artery. At present most procedures utilize a metallic stent that was found more efficient and durable.

Unfortunately, sudden death can sometimes be the first presentation. However, later interviews with patients whose lives were saved by prompt intervention and resuscitation often reveal that they had indeed suffered from some chest discomfort prior to the event which they didn't consider as being serious. Other manifestations include shortness of breath, palpitations, and fainting.

In summary, the disease may declare itself with typical chest pain or it can be more insidious and treacherous, striking dramatically with sudden collapse. This explains why many victims will not even make it to the hospital. The severity of arterial narrowing is not the sole predictor of upcoming serious events. Composition of the plaque and certain other chemicals formed into the inside linings (endothelium) of arteries - as well as active substances and stress hormones - all play a major role in determining the course toward instability or potential complications. Paradoxically, blockages that are only moderately severe can lead to more heart attacks, especially in younger individuals, than severe and calcified blockages in older ones. Mortality from heart attacks remains quite high and the majority of deaths occur before reaching a hospital.

Establishing The Diagnosis *What's going on?*

Apart from emergency cases, treatment should not be initiated until some confirmatory evidence of the disease is at hand. Typical symptoms as in the case of Ms. Vera Santos help raise the index of suspicion. Physical examination usually falls short of proving the existence of disease, let alone its severity. A simple test utilizing the time honored Electrocardiographic recording (ECG) at the time of physical pain may show highly specific signs effectively revealing the diagnosis. Otherwise a "stress test" would be recommended. A graded treadmill exercise test according to pre-set protocol of gradual acceleration may unveil signs of ischemia by the depression of a line called ST. Segment. Further confirmation can be obtained by **nuclear imaging test** utilizing intravenous injection of a nuclear tracer called Thallium that has high affinity to heart muscle. Subsequent camera obtained images show, in case of ischemia, a reduction of the tracer concentrations in areas of the heart lacking adequate blood supply, indirectly suggesting the presence of stenosed (narrowed) arteries. In people who are physically unable to perform exercise (due to incapacity, old age, or physical disability) the test can be done after an injection of a chemical called dipyridamol (persantin), which simulates the effect of physical exercise. Another somewhat simpler test called **Stress Echocardiogram** reflects a reduction of motion function in the affected areas of heart muscle as seen on an ultrasound recording at the peak of an exercise test. If the patient cannot perform exercise, recording can be made after intravenous infusion of a cardiac muscle stimulating drug called Dobutamine. The gold standard test of Coronary Cineangiography would probably be recommended if the above tests are abnormal (or positive). This test is done by direct injection of a contrast media into the coronary arteries, via fine tubes (catheters) inserted into arteries in the legs or arms. This test allows for not only a clear visualization of the narrowed area of an artery, but also a measure of how severe it is. The procedure provides avenues for subsequent treatments with angioplasty methods if these are judged to be necessary, and can be performed as an extension of the same procedure.

Management Of Coronary Heart Disease
Or how to "Hold the Bull by the Horns"

Once the presence of the disease is established, multiple modalities of treatment may be found helpful or necessary. Drugs are essential and include compounds that dilate the arteries, such as **nitroglycerine,** which can abort the pain of angina attacks. Others work by reducing the heart muscle demand for oxygen by decreasing heart rate and force of contractility, such as the class of drugs called **beta blockers.** Cholesterol-lowering drugs—including the compounds known as Statins, Fibrates and Nicotinic acid—are needed in patients suffering from Lipid disorders. Another group of drugs that prevent blood platelets from forming clots is highlighted by the time proven **Aspirin,** which can be very helpful. In many patients, especially those with implanted coronary artery stents, additional Antiplatelets power may be needed. This includes a drug called Clopidogrel (Plavix). If medications fail to control symptoms, more aggressive and invasive treatments may be required. These include balloon dilatation of the narrowed segments and placement of metal stents utilizing the technique of catheterization, called Percutaneous Coronary Intervention (PCI). Should this technique prove to be inadequate or too complex to perform and therefore more risky, then coronary bypass operation may become necessary. Utilizing pieces of veins removed from a patient's legs, or arteries removed from their arms or the inside of their chests, a bridge is constructed around the blocked area to function as a virtual "detour".

Fortunately today many such operations can be performed while the chest is open and the heart is still beating. This seems to reduce the rate of surgical complications in comparison with the traditional approach of arresting the heart and diverting the circulation. Most recently, utilizing a robotic computer - controlled arm, the surgeon can operate through much smaller chest incisions.

Prevention of coronary artery disease, once a mere dream, seems to be more effective than ever before. Optimism is mounting as it becomes apparent that the death rate and the number of new cases are on the decline. The adoption of healthier life styles certainly deserves major credit, including more balanced eating habits, exercise, weight reduction, and control of stress. Unfortunately, definitive success of these programs remains hard to achieve since it requires unrelenting commitment and adherence. The role of public education led by professional heart organizations and leading academic centers is pivotal and seems to have had a significant impact on motivating those affected with multiple risk factors. Prevention campaigns are especially challenging for the many people suffering from the so-called Metabolic Syndrome.* Resistance to naturally secreted insulin hormone seems to be associated not only with diabetes but also with high levels of cholesterol and lipids, high blood pressure, obesity and even tendencies for clot formations. All these factors can work in concert to induce the arterial disease leading to heart attacks. Naturally, more concentrated efforts are needed in this group of patients and, hopefully, new drugs and treatments effective in breaking this vicious cycle are on the way. In the San Francisco Bay area, where I practice, the metabolic syndrome seems to be especially common amongst the immigrant population, in particular those coming from eastern countries and the Pacific Islands. Any breakthrough in prevention and treatment would come as a result of combined efforts by the health authorities, the media, and community institutions and its leaders.

It remains to be established whether medical management and lifestyle changes can prevent the formation or slow the buildup of plaque in the arteries. Recurrence of ischemia and re-occlusion in previously dilated or bypassed arteries, or in the bypass conduits themselves, may require the repetition of interventional procedures.

Even with advanced disease, continuation of preventive measures—known as secondary prevention—remains essential for a satisfactory

---

* A syndrome is a collection of clinical manifestations that fit into one scheme or form a recognizable entity.

8

outcome. Here, the drug groups—called Statins—and other lipid lowering agents, as well as stricter life style modifications, play a major role. In addition, a daily dose of aspirin and beta blocking drugs and absolute discontinuation of cigarette smoking are of utmost importance.

Q. What does the future hold?
A: A lot!

The final battle against coronary heart disease will most likely be won not by intervention but rather by prevention. In the meantime, more advanced technologies are being used to re-establish blood flow in blocked arteries as soon as possible after the onset or during the course of a heart attack. Potent "clot busters" such as TPA and the Kinase enzymes were successfully used in many cases with surprisingly low chance of bleeding complications. Drugs that paralyze platelet activity are commonly used in conjunction with mechanical intervention. Stents that release chemicals to prevent the formation of scar tissue—which can eventually re-occlude the stent itself—are now extensively used worldwide.*

More perfected devices and drugs are being investigated. Thus far, the role of laser technology has not taken hold but is still not totally shelved. In many patients, coronary bypass surgery is the treatment of choice. This is especially true for widespread disease affecting multiple arterial branches or blockages located in critical areas rendering non-surgical interventions risky. The majority of these operations are now performed without having to arrest the heart function and divert the circulation. The use of a natural artery in the front of the chest cavity, called the internal mammary artery, as a bypass has been proven to be extremely effective as a long-term treatment, largely due to its not yet fully understood resistance to blockage. So far there is no proven effective bypass conduit made from synthetic material even though these conduits are quite useful in arteries that are much larger than the coronary arteries.

Studies are constantly being designed and performed to establish the indications, limitations, and risks of all these therapeutic modalities. As experience and knowledge increase, the results of interventions are progressively improving. Bypass operations in Octogenarians (over the

---

* These devices are referred to as drug eluting stents. Recently, late occlusion was recognized to occur. Continuation of antiplatelets drugs such as Clopidogrel is now considered imperative.

age of 80 years) are now routinely performed with surprisingly low risk.

Genetic science and heart disease is still in the infancy stage. Major heart research centers seem to be committed to advancement and they continue to explore this domain. Early return involves identification of genetic markers for several heart disease conditions. Therapeutic applications may hold significant promise in the future.

The area that seems to be getting "hotter" involves stem cell research. This may prove to be valuable for the treatment of conditions characterized by heart enlargement and progressive weakening of its pumping function, leading to severe heart failure. Early experimental studies are raising hopes that adult stem cells can be used to repair the widespread damage in the heart muscle and actually promote an improvement in mechanical heart function, eventually reducing the need for heart transplant operations.

CHAPTER TWO

HEART MUSCLE DISEASE

The coronary arteries are fine, but the heart muscle is not and can actually become very sick.

HEART MUSCLE DISEASE (CARDIOMYOPATHY)

Can the heart muscle get sick in the absence of blockages of the arteries?

"It's All In The Family"

John Colder was only twenty-five years old when new symptoms lead to the suspicion that he might have a serious heart condition. He was not at all surprised and told me that he had been waiting to hear this for many years. He told me about his older brother whose heart had completely failed prompting him to have heart transplant as an only option. John knew all along that his brother was suffering from a condition called **Familial Cardiomyopathy** and that he himself was under risk. Being the brave young man he was, he decided to remain resilient and fight back. Despair and surrender were not part of his nature. He was told that the echocardiogram* showed his heart to be much larger and weaker than the results of the same test two years earlier. The following week, John was already taking five different medications. New discoveries have worked in his favor. Research has found that a cocktail of drugs, including Beta Blockers, Angiotensin Receptors Blockers, Spironolactone in addition to traditional heart failure drugs (such as diuretics and Digoxin) can slow the progression of heart weakness. John could live in comfort, provided he took his medications without

---

* Echocardiogram: ultrasound recording that accurately detects and estimates severity of heart enlargement and weakness.

13

interruption. He later required a procedure to implant a special device - Pacemaker Defibrillator, which made him feel even better. Short of heart catheterization, no other operation was needed. John knew he was to live the rest of his life on guard for any undesirable sign or test result threatening recurrence of his heart disease. He was so happy that both he and his brother had benefited, in different ways, from modern medicine. Medical advancement helped arrest their otherwise deadly condition.

The medical term cardiomyopathy denotes a group of conditions of variable causes that share two cardinal features:

First, they all affect the heart muscle directly—**not** by means of altering the blood supply to the heart or diseased heart valves.

Second, reversing or modifying the underlying cause at an early phase can improve the outlook. Full or partial recovery can occur spontaneously or as a result of special treatments or interventions. Once irreversible damage occurs—due to widespread scarring of the heart muscle—the condition becomes incurable, frequently leading to disability or death. In the majority of such cases the myocardium loses much of its pumping and/or relaxation functions.* The heart becomes unable to adequately provide enough blood and, therefore, to deliver oxygen to working organs and tissues throughout the body.

The physician would commonly inform the affected patient that his or her heart is enlarged and very weak and that the arteries and valves are not much affected. Certain tests are frequently performed, including ultrasound recordings called "echocardiogram," which can clearly show the enlargement of heart chambers and assess the severity of reduced function. Occasionally heart catheterization and imaging with contrast material (angiogram) or even taking a biopsy of the heart muscle may be required to establish the diagnosis and find the possible underlying cause.

Cardiomyopathies are usually viewed as two different types. In the first, heart chambers, especially the main pumping chamber (left ventricle), are dilated and their muscular walls thinned out with very poor pumping action. Conversely, the second type is characterized by very thick muscle with preservation of the pumping power that can even be hyperactive. While this may look good on the surface, it is not necessarily the case. The walls of the chamber may become stiff and unable to sufficiently relax during the filling phase to accommodate the needed

---

* Pumping function: heart muscle ability to contract and squeeze blood out of the chamber. Relaxation function is the ability to relax and allow incoming blood to fill the cavity.

volume of blood. The pump filling is therefore not optimal, thus the output is reduced. This can become even more complicated if the part of the muscle surrounding the area where blood exits from the heart becomes so thick that it can limit the flow of blood out of the heart. This less common type is called obstructive and can cause serious consequences ranging from simple fainting to sudden death. This latter extreme event has been identified as one of a few underlying causes of tragic and dramatic death in seemingly healthy people, including athletes in the midst of high-energy games.

Back to emotions...

Can emotional stress cause cardiomyopathy without demonstrable coronary artery disease? After all, the Broken Heart syndrome is but an acute form of cardiomyopathy induced by the outpouring of stress hormones. Should the emotional trauma become repetitive or the stress sustained, an ongoing or chronic form of cardiomyopathy may result. Furthermore, repeated bouts of depression can also adversely affect the heart performance.

What Can Weaken A Heart That Much?

Many causes of heart muscle disease have been identified while others remain enigmatic. In modern societies, coronary heart disease is the number one cause of damage to the heart muscle. This is often referred to as Ischemic Heart Disease". The list of causes of heart muscle disease keeps growing. Emotional heart disease generally termed "stress cardiomyopathy" is but the latest addition. A few conditions usually called primary cardiomyopathy affect only the heart muscle and cause either enlargement (dilatation) of the chambers or increased thickness of their walls (hypertrophy). Many of these cases are genetically determined and tend to run in members of the same family. The others are a variety of general medical illnesses that involve the heart muscle among other body organs and tissues. Examples of this include:

1. Invasion of the heart muscle by a material called Amyloid as part of a generalized disorder, which limits the ability of the heart muscle to relax and accept the incoming blood to fill its chambers.
2. Collagen Vascular Disease: this is an umbrella name for a still elusive illness such as lupus, or rheumatoid arthritis. The culprit is a

mysterious vascular inflammation in which the body's immune system seems to turn against its own organs, including the heart.

3. Alcoholic heart disease, due to direct toxicity from alcohol abuse causing heart enlargement and failure, a condition called Alcoholic Cardiomyopathy.

4. Involvement of the heart muscle by a certain Viral Infection (the common virus is from a group named Coxackie, usually a cause of respiratory infections.

5. Direct toxicity of an unknown cause that occurs in late pregnancy and the period after delivery, usually labeled Post-Partum Cardiomyopathy. The condition tends to get worse with subsequent pregnancies.

6. Chagas Disease, common in South America, is caused by a parasite and selectively affects the heart muscle.

7. Drug abuse or addiction is a growing cause, especially in young individuals. Methamphetamine and cocaine top the list of drugs that are toxic to the heart muscle. Certain drugs used in cancer chemotherapy are also implicated.

MANAGEMENT
How to Reenergize a Tired Horse:

The treatment of heart muscle disease (the Cardiomyopathies) is understandably very complex, in view of the several different ways they alter heart function. A medicine that can be helpful in one type can be harmful in another. Familial types, especially the hypertrophic variety, are compatible with long life and are often discovered in the elderly. When heart failure symptoms such as shortness of breath, fatigue, palpitations, leg swelling, or fainting spells appear, prompt and often aggressive treatment becomes mandatory. Frequent hospital admissions are common and typically, multiple medications are used. These include diuretics, to help enhance the kidney's removal of excessive retained fluid, and others to improve the pumping power of the heart muscle, or to treat heart rhythm disturbances since either fast or slow heart rate can adversely affect the function. A group of drugs called beta blockers were found to be quite helpful to many patients by intercepting the often excessive outpouring of stress hormones. Intended by the body as a rallying effort to assist the failing heart and keep the blood pressure from falling, they can overwhelm the already very weak muscle and make it even weaker. In other words, it doesn't help to "keep whipping an exhausted horse!"

If medical treatment appears to be failing, new electronic pacemaker devices can provide additional help. They are programmed to stimulate both the right and left pumping chambers and better synchronize their actions, adding more efficiency with improved output. In advanced heart failure, sudden death, due to heart fibrillation, is fairly common. A device now well known to the public, called defibrillator, is increasingly implanted in high risk patients to deliver an electric shock as needed to reset the heart into regular rhythm. Nowadays, these devices are often incorporated with the pacemakers into one system.

What can be done should all the above measures fail or fall short of supporting a meaningful life style? The answer is heart transplantation. This is an effective but seriously complex treatment constrained by the need for rigorous follow up care, but more significantly, hindered by the limited availability of donor hearts. In order to overcome these two major shortcomings, research is at earnest to produce more practical artificial devices to replace the human heart altogether. On a separate track, scientists have been able to grow healthy heart muscle tissue, by utilizing stem cell technology, hoping to someday use it to support the failing heart or even replace it. Reports describing the progress of this innovation are generating much excitement in medical circles and are also triggering a glimpse of hope for the many unfortunate people whose hearts have already shown a very limited ability to keep on beating.

CHAPTER THREE

THE EARLY EVIDENCE OF EMOTIONAL HEART DISEASE

EUREKA!!

SPASM OF CORONARY ARTERIES
The Finding of a "Missing Link"

The Story OF A BROKEN HEART:

For 62 year old Margaret, her dream of a happy peaceful life was supposed to have already been realized. Instead, her troubles seem to have just begun. Her husband, five years her senior, had become an alcoholic and lost most of his reasoning. To prove his dominance he started battering her and threatening her with divorce.. Her only source of pleasure was a granddaughter, Sally. A strong loving bond had developed between the two. Margaret had all but forgotten her former dreams of traveling around the world, or relaxing at a luxurious spa. She settled to live for the young girl, who she watched grow up into a beautiful teenager of thirteen. She often stated that the young girl was her only reason to live. This is why when Sally was kidnapped and raped, Margaret suffered the most profound shock of her life. She started experiencing tight chest pains and breathing difficulty. Initial medical evaluation was suggestive of coronary artery disease with angina and "stuttering" heart attack. A twenty four hour heart monitor placed on her chest showed marked changes occurring during the pain and indicative of profound heart muscle ischemia. The next step was coronary angiography. During the procedure she suffered from another episode of chest pain. Simultaneous angiographic recording showed severe spasm of a large heart artery constricting its lumen to over eighty percent. Administration of nitroglycerine relieved both the pain and the artery spasm. Margaret's life would never be the same again. With very little left to lose, she estranged herself, but maintained her medical care and an even more loving attachment to her granddaughter Sally.

A MEDICAL MYSTERY

Over the past century, thanks to the objective scientific approach, many of the mysteries of heart disease have been unlocked or at least reasonably understood. However, many others remain quite elusive. Cardinal among these has been the occurrence of angina, and even heart attacks, in the absence of any demonstrable coronary artery disease. Let us first learn about the traditional form of angina:

Classic or "HEBERDEN" Angina*

Heberden's classic description of angina over two hundred years ago has until recently dominated both the clinical diagnosis of ischemia as well as the understanding of the mechanisms involved. The increase in the demand for oxygen during exercise coupled with a supply limited by a narrowed artery can result in the onset of anginal pain. In a typical episode, the patient describes having oppressive discomfort, commonly localized in mid chest area and often radiating to the upper chest, neck, jaws, upper back, and forearms especially the left side. The patient typically expresses the constricting nature of the pain by making a fist with his hand and then placing it in the middle of his chest. This historical "fist sign" still retains, nowadays, a major diagnostic significance. The pain is usually relieved a few minutes after resting or placing a nitroglycerine pill under the tongue. However, if the pain persists or continues to build up, a heart attack may be eminent. The patient, following his physician's advice, would call 911 for help. A well-equipped paramedic ambulance is usually dispatched and the patient will most probably end up in a hospital emergency room for confirmation of diagnosis and further treatment. Simulation of the above presentation is often portrayed in movies or television programs such as "ER" and "House," and has helped to popularize a basic awareness of this condition among the public at large.

---

* Angina: constricting pain in the front of the chest due to inadequate blood supply to the heart muscle, as a result of diseased coronary arteries.

Can "ischemia" be silent or more precisely painless?
"A silent Killer"

The answer is yes. Indeed serious episodes of ischemia and even heart attacks may not be associated with pain. However, the majority of these are signaled by other symptoms of equivalent significance such as "heart burn", breathing difficulty, nausea, arm discomfort, or sensation of irregular heart beat. Truly silent episodes or at least ignorable by the patient can occur especially in sufferers of diabetes or certain disorders of the neurological system.

Occasionally, patients may mistakenly relate their symptom to "indigestion" or "acid reflux". Surprisingly, even well-informed physicians, including cardiologists driven by denial, may ignore their own symptoms and miss an opportunity for early treatment. Not infrequently, scarred areas of previous heart attacks are discovered by electrocardiograms or echocardiograms in patients who cannot recall having had any chest pain, or may vaguely recall having unpleasant discomfort in the chest area.

STABLE AND UNSTABLE ANGINA:
"A Cold War and a Hot War"

The theory of increased demand that overwhelms the ability to augment supply can explain most anginal pain occurring only after effort. Predictability of the level (threshold) of effort needed to incite pain and how to terminate it are also signs of stability thus the name "stable angina". New disruptions in the anatomy of the plaque* that further compromise the lumen size, or interference of other external forces such as rapid heart action, anxiety, or certain medications, may temporarily or permanently change this balance. Many patients with stable angina can be treated medically. In addition, some studies found no real added benefit from interventional treatment with multiple stents, especially in the elderly. On the contrary, unstable angina usually means an "active plaque" within the artery, often complicated by a break (fissure) and clot formation. Disruption of the layer of cells lining the inside of the artery—called the endothelium—results in the release of powerful sub-

---

* Plaque: is a raised patch composed of lipids such as cholesterol as well as fibers and certain types of cells. A large plaque can partially obstruct the artery. Total blockage can result if the plaque breaks and a blood clot is formed.

stances including one called "Endothelin" that can cause new problems by constricting the artery with further reduction of blood flow. In addition, a healthy endothelial cell is essential for maintaining blood flow also by secreting a substance called The Endothelium - Derived Relaxing Factor (EDRF), that helps to maintain the compliance of the arterial wall and keep it open. Additionally a certain type of active blood cells called platelets play a role in this process within the artery. Normally helpful to control bleeding by forming a "white clot" at the site, they can suddenly be turned on and become active. This produces a substance called Thromboxane A2 (TXA2), a potent stimulator of platelet clogging and arterial constriction. Eventually this raging "hot war" can lead to total occlusion of the artery and the beginning of a heart attack with its well-known consequences, including heart failure, abnormal heart rhythm, and sudden death. The very important function of the arterial wall has become more evident. Constriction (spasm) or relaxation (dilatation) may occur during the course of ischemia. This concept was first raised by Latham, in the late nineteenth century, and then by Osler, in the early twentieth century. These alterations in vascular tones are crucially important in the induction of ischemia and the understanding of the connection between coronary artery spasm and emotional reactions, the subject of this book. In order to begin to understand, we must address the concept of how spasm can occur in an apparently normal artery and cause angina, not by increasing demand, but rather by reducing supply.

VARIANT ANGINA: *"The other angina"*

The hallmark of this atypical form of angina is its occurrence without effort and association with changes on the electrocardiogram that simulate an early myocardial infarction (heart attack). All other features are shared with classic angina including the quality of chest pain and relief after administration of nitroglycerine. This syndrome, first described by Prinzmetal in 1959, was found to be associated with severe narrowing of the corresponding coronary artery. The proposed mechanism suggests that superimposed spasm* results in temporary total occlusion, not unlike that found in an acute heart attack. Relief of

---

* Spasm of an artery denotes a usually reversible constriction that can reduce the inside lumen to a variable degree. Spasm results mostly from increased tone of the arterial wall commonly due to sympathetic nerve stimulation or chemicals released from the endothelial cells in the artery itself. Stress Hormones are also capable of doing the same

the spasm by nitroglycerine may indeed inhibit progression into true heart attack.

In 1973, I was working with a team of cardiologists at George Washington University. We described an identical syndrome with one exception: the coronary arteries were normal on angiogram. Spasm was postulated and indeed documented in several patients. We characterized this new syndrome as a "variant of the variant." At the time of these striking observations, emotional history was not sought. However, since then a link with traumatic emotional experience has been strongly suspected. Catecholamine hormones were presumed to be the mediators.

EMOTIONS, *The Other Missing Link*

Can spasm induced by substances such as catecholamine hormones represent the missing link that determines stability and instability of the angina syndrome? And if this is indeed the case, can emotional trauma serve as the trigger mechanism for heart attacks? Indirect evidence has since surfaced revealing the not infrequent occurrence of heart attacks due to complete closure of arteries that were previously narrowed to only sixty percent or less of their lumen size.

Therefore, the mechanism may not be simply progressive narrowing to the point of complete blockage, but an acute disruption triggering interplay of spasm and active chemical substances working in concert to eventually completely block the artery by clot formation.

More recent observations have shed some light on arteries prone to spasm. While appearing perfectly clean on angiograms, they are actually not. A certain degree of early atherosclerotic changes are usually present and may well be a prerequisite for spasm. External stimuli such as emotional trauma may then work in concert with an endothelium layer altered by atherosclerosis to promote spasm mediated by local substances. How essential or decisive the role of emotional stress in triggering the above events is now the subject of further scientific investigation. As will be discussed later in detail, the observation of cardiac crisis occurring subsequent to emotional trauma is hardly debatable nowadays. What needs to be established is basically how essential is the role of the emotional trigger. Subacute but ongoing, unresolved stress can also result in heart muscle damage in a more indiscrete and frequently unrecognizable manner. In general, it is assumed that unvented stress may be more harmful than that displayed by variable expressions such as outbursts of anger or grief.

The value of incorporating neuroscience with heart disease research is clearly important. The unknown but suspected aspects of a brain-heart connection are too extensive and important to ignore.

So far we have in this chapter gone through aspects of heart disease that are essential in order to build up the case for what can be called emotional heart disease. Next and equally important is to know more about the science of emotions where startling revelations have already emerged and more work is continuing at earnest. This is the subject of the next chapter.

CHAPTER FOUR

HUMAN EMOTIONS

Probably the most complex
phenomenon on the planet

Human emotions may well be the most complex phenomenon on our planet. Research on emotions has been hampered by the lack of a basic "alphabet," making coordinated research rather difficult. In other words, the building blocks of human emotions were not identified until the last century. This is not to suggest that emotions were not experienced by early humans or later by the clusters of societies that eventually transformed into civilizations. On the contrary, profound emotional experiences have influenced the activities of individuals and the masses for millennia. Indeed emotions have determined the course of the world, leading to war or peace throughout known history. To illustrate the power of emotions over human behavior, I will dedicate the following pages to recounting stories of epic proportions that were fueled by domineering emotions.

SELECTED EPICS OF EMOTIONS IN HISTORY
AND
IN LITERATURE

Both factual history and legend based fictional literature have produced a wealth of recounts of love, hatred, jealousy, hostility, revenge and many other manifestations of heightened human emotions. In many instances, the powers embodied in these feelings have lead to marvelous construction. In other instances, these feelings have brought about ominous destruction. This helps us to understand the "positive" and the "negative" aspects of uncontrolled emotions. Lovers as well as conquerors have been revered by the masses for setting examples of bravery or sacrifice for the generations that followed. The intensity of the emotionally based struggles in some of these accounts is but a reflection of the power of the underlying emotion. Much of history was either driven or profoundly influenced by emotions experienced by leaders and the masses in both sides of any conflict, truce, or alliance.

Highlights of five such epics are presented in the following pages.

LOVING THE ENEMY: *Aida*
(from Giuseppe Verdi's Opera)

This Ethiopian princess, who was enslaved in Egypt, guarded her secret love for Radames, the Egyptian commander who invaded her country and captured her own beloved father. Torn between her love for Radames, her love for her father, and loyalty to her country she managed to keep all. From his side, Radames denounced all the glory of victory bestowed upon him by the Pharaoh including an arranged marriage to the Pharaoh's daughter Amneris, who was also secretly in love with Radames. Radames made it clear that Aida was the one he wanted to marry; yet, when his conspiracy with her and her father to flee was uncovered, his honor led him to surrender and face condemnation to death. The power of love reached a climax when Aida having seen the great sacrifices of her lover, opted to hide herself in the vault where Radames was later lead to before it was sealed. She decided to die with Radames. The two lovers accepted their fate together.

The capacity to love the conqueror of her country represents indeed a new dimension of love. The predominantly fictional nature of this story does not in any way reduce the emotional credential, which is the human fiber of this fable.

ETERNAL HOSTILITY & VENGEANCE:
Hannibal Of Carthage

Hostility and vengeance are two potent complex emotions that empowered great leaders and motivated them during events that have reverberated throughout human history.

The Carthaginian general Hannibal (247-182 BC) waged wars and accomplished conquests, making him one of the greatest military leaders in history. He was the eldest son of a powerful Carthaginian general who lost the first Punic War to the Romans. The young Hannibal would never forget the humiliation his father suffered as the Romans stripped Carthage of its most valuable provinces. At the age of ten, he moved to Iberia (today's Spain) where Carthaginians had succeeded in expanding their influence with the bustling cities of Cadiz, Malaga, and Cartagena.

Inspired by this success, young Hannibal began his march against his father's enemies: the Romans. He had promised his eternal hatred of the Romans to his father and with it his unrelenting drive to avenge the defeat of the first Punic War. Hannibal teamed up with new friends—the Gaul's—who shared his hatred of the Romans. The Gauls, recently subjugated to Rome, were very willing to help Hannibal bring an end to Rome's iron fisted control. Hannibal's army of fifty thousand men was met by eighty thousand Roman soldiers. And still, Hannibal and his allies toasted a victory over Rome. Capua became Hannibal's capital in Italy.

In time, Carthage was forced to recall its army and to leave Italy after a succession of Roman achievements. After a final battle with Scipio at Zama, Hannibal had to escape to Carthage in humiliation. But he was not to abandon his dream of conquering Rome. Being the great commander that he was, he resorted to tactical negotiations with the Romans to conclude a peace treaty, under humiliating terms. It was his only option to survive and plot a comeback to pursue his passionate dream of revenge.

This time around Hannibal changed tactics, trying to ally Carthage with the massive Seleucid Empire under Antiochus III the Great whom he tried to convince to invade Rome presumably with himself as the commander. Antiochus was pre-occupied at the time with an invasion of Greece to stall Rome's expansionism and establish a zone of influence in Greece. For the Seleucid King this was both more important and achievable. He already had a great empire extending through Anatolia, Syria, Mesopotamia, and Persia. Unlike Hannibal, he did not have the passion to sacrifice everything in order to destroy Rome. Nevertheless, Antiochus Ill lost his war with Rome over Greece and Macedonia. This allowed the small kingdom of Pergamon, allied with Rome, to take over today's Turkey. As long as he was alive, Hannibal was never to abandon the passion that had totally overtaken him. He made an attempt helping a separatist Seleucid governor to establish a kingdom in today's Armenia. When this did not promote his dream, he supported Bithynia in a war against Pergamon where he achieved his final military victory. When mighty Rome came to the rescue, Hannibal realized that his great power and determination for revenge had all come to an end. He accepted his fate and in order to avoid humiliation, he was reported to have poisoned himself.

AN EPIC OF LOVE AND HATRED:
Romeo and Juliet

This story of love and hatred as told by William Shakespeare has captured the hearts of the young and the old for generations. Just like a beautiful lily growing from the trash, the love between Romeo and Juliet blossomed despite ancient hatred and quarrels between their two families. Regardless of whether the foundation of this story is legend or real, there is no doubt that it represents true emotions of people everywhere. In fact, only recently, the skeletons of a young man and a young woman, apparently lovers embracing each other, were unearthed near the city of Mantua where Romeo, according to the story, was exiled. Could it be that legends of these two or other lovers survived to be retold later? Could an emotional experience born in the imagination of a novelist indeed represent true events experienced by real people?

Romeo, a Montague, fell in love with Juliet, a Capulet. The two families had turned a lovely town called Verona into a battlefield reflecting their hatred of one another. The intrusion of Romeo into a Capulet party inflamed a young Capulet named Tybalt who intended to kill Romeo and ended up killing Mercutio, Romeo's friend, only to be killed himself by Romeo, acting in self defense. The two lovers managed to meet in secret and even spend a full night together before Romeo had to flee to Mantua. Friar Lawrence who earlier performed a marriage ceremony for Romeo and Juliet tried to help Juliet. He wanted to spoil a plan that would force Juliet to marry a young prince named Paris. He gave her a potion that would have her appear dead for two days, and then sent a message to Romeo informing him of the plan. Romeo never received the message and hearing of Juliet's "death", he rushed to the vault and took a poison to die hugging and kissing her. When Juliet awoke and found Romeo dead she took her own life, stabbing herself with his dagger. "For without Romeo she did not wish to live." The sacrifice of the two lovers brought the two warring families to end their historic mutual hatred and to live amicably. The love between a man and a woman, as the story's moral suggests, can only grow stronger when met with obstacles. In the meantime, it can arouse hatred in the hearts of opponents.

POWER AND LUST:
Cleopatra of Egypt

Desire to hold absolute power to control everyone and own everything may well be the ultimate in the complex human emotions. Throughout history, there have only been a few supreme rulers to reach this level of emotional disturbance of greed and yearning for absolute dominance. Cleopatra, the last Pharaoh of Egypt, ranks high on this list. Her reign marked a transition between the Hellenistic era established by Ptolemy I, one of the generals of Alexander the Great, and the Roman dominated era. Cleopatra's culture was predominantly Hellenistic despite a formal preservation, of the Egyptian belief system of gods and goddesses, including her patron goddess of wisdom Isis, of whom she was considered to be a re-incarnation. Through liaisons with Julius Caesar and his successor Mark Antony, Cleopatra was able to solidify her grasp on the throne of the Pharaohs for over 20 years, from 51 BC to 30 BC.

Her ascension to the throne ended a sequence of violence within the Royal family probably unprecedented in history. Both her elder sisters attempted to seize power one after the other, only to be executed leaving Cleopatra as the likely heiress. After her father Ptolemy XII died, she shared power with a younger brother. Her enterprise to gain exclusive power and isolate her brother later backfired as a palace rebellion declared her brother, Ptolemy, sole ruler. Cleopatra was forced into exile, only to find another chance to regain power as Julius Caesar, the victor of Roman civil war, arrived in Alexandria with a plan to annex Egypt Against the might of Caesar, Cleopatra used her last weapon, the power of seduction.

Julius Caesar was so charmed by her enticing gestures that nine months after their meeting, Cleopatra gave birth to their son Caesarion. Caesar at this point decided to preserve the Egyptian throne and restore his now official lover Cleopatra as the Queen of Egypt. However, the limit of her influence on him became apparent by his refusal to name Caesarion his son from Cleopatra as his heir, a move that would have united Rome and Egypt under one ruler. In a ruthless drive to maintain her power and secure the throne for her son, Cleopatra arranged to have her only living sister killed.

A new chapter in Cleopatra's zeal for power was to begin after Julius Caesar was assassinated. A new liaison was forged with Mark Anthony, the successor of Julius Caesar. Like Julius, Mark Anthony was captivated by her charm. After a winter in Alexandria, their love affair resulted in the birth of twins, a boy and a girl. Later Anthony made Alexandria his home and Cleopatra his wife. The marriage produced four more children. In 34 BC three of their children were crowned as rulers of different Mediterranean and Near Eastern Provinces and Cleopatra was named Queen of Kings. A life marked by greed, lust, and ruthlessness is unlikely to lead to a safe haven. Despite her legendary skills and magnetism of an incredible durability, Cleopatra was heading for yet another, and this time fateful, upheaval. The Romans were outraged by Anthony's behavior prompting the senate to authorize Octavian to invade Egypt In the ensuing Naval battle, the forces of Anthony and Cleopatra proved not to be a match for the Roman fleet. Cleopatra fled and Anthony abandoned the battle seemingly to follow her. The accounts regarding the final chapter are varied; however, there seems to be a general agreement that the two lovers had spent their final hours together. The most dramatic version suggests that Cleopatra, fearing the wrath of Anthony who allegedly accused her of betrayal, locked herself in her room with two servants. Anthony, hearing that she died, stabbed himself but survived. He later joined Cleopatra only to die in her arms. Most historians believe that Cleopatra ended her life by allowing two Asps to bite her.

The immense dimension of a real historical chronicle that dealt with intense human passions of powerful historical figures has all contributed to the everlasting interest of this story over the generations. Two literary masters have eternalized these events, William Shakespeare in "Anthony and Cleopatra" and George Bernard Shaw in "Caesar and Cleopatra".

LOVING TO ADORATION:
Taj Mahal

The love of Emperor Shah Jahan (1592-1666), the Mughal Emperor of India, for his Queen Mumtaz Mahal, reaches legendary proportions. It was said that just like lovebirds, he teetered on the brink of death after she died. His passionate love for her was ignited at an early age: he was sixteen, she was fifteen. Despite her aristocratic upbringing, being the daughter of a powerful prime minister, she was extremely kind, humble and loving, and of course, stunningly beautiful. Her name then was Arjumand and his was Khurram.

The young man, who had already accomplished high skills in battle, music and architecture, asked his father Emperor Jahangir to bless his wish to marry Arjumand. After five years of not being allowed to see each other, the long awaited marriage was officially consummated. The new Queen was renamed Mumtaz Mahal and her husband ascended to the throne as Emperor Shah Jahan. The Emperor's love for his queen grew even stronger as she blossomed into a very intelligent and compassionate woman. After seven children together, the Queen was pregnant again; meanwhile, her husband was engaged in a war with his enemy Jahan Lodi.

After delivering the baby, Mumtaz died. The shock of her death was too much for the emperor to bear. For eight days, he locked himself in total isolation—moaning constantly, refusing to eat or meet with anyone. He even expressed his desire to renounce all his power and live a simple life thriving only on her memory. He committed himself to build for his beloved queen the most splendid monument ever built as an expression of love of a man for a woman. The mausoleum named "Taj Mahal" stands out nowadays as one of the most serene and beautiful structures in the world. To this day it remains a symbol of love ascending to adoration.

EVOLVING CONCEPTS ON HUMAN EMOTIONS

Human emotional activity has been, for centuries, unfairly and mistakenly separated from science. Moreover, emotions have been frequently viewed as anti-science. Emotional reactions are thought to drive human intellect away from reality and objectivity. Some aspects of this logic are understandable since overreaction can distract from recognition of facts that are at times hard to accept or to even face. The lack of understanding of the physiology of emotions has given rise to certain taboos that view emotions as a form of primitive or somehow inferior level of behavior. The revolutionary rise of neuroscience over the last century has all but changed the way we deal with emotions, which are viewed nowadays as a normal and natural activity stemming from the interaction between the mind and the brain. Calling neuroscience the "last frontier" in human and medical sciences no longer seems fantastical or an exaggeration.

While major concepts and discoveries continue to emerge in the field of physical and space sciences, there has been a relative recession in medical frontiers. The only exception to this is neuroscience, where major revelations and concepts are already on the horizon and are expected to radically change the way we think and live. The relationship between the mind, sometimes viewed as the "soul", and the brain as an organ occupies the centerfold of an ever expanding wealth of knowledge. The subject is stirring more interest thanks to heated debates within the realms of medicine, philosophy, and psychosocial science.

The basic argument is centered on whether the mind is a product of the brain machine, fully controlled by the higher brain centers, or, is it simply a software program, running on the brain-computer?

Within the scope of this book we are mostly interested in the impact of emotional activity on the function of organ systems, especially the heart. But before we come to that, we would be empowered by a basic understanding of the science of emotions.

BASIC EMOTIONS:

The action and interaction of basic emotions play a fundamental role in characterizing the personality of any given individual. There is a general consensus between most neuroscientists that at least six basic emotions are now identifiable: fear, joy, sadness, anger, disgust, and surprise. Either one can be profound enough to stir a quake of metabolic changes ignited by a host of stress hormones and neurotransmitters. Depending on the nature and the intensity and rapidity of the reaction, it can exert a considerable impact on the function as well as the structural integrity of the heart, the circulation and probably several other organ systems.

CAN EMOTIONS BE CLASSIFIED?

A simplistic, and probably also realistic, way is to view human emotions, despite their many diversities, as a continuum, stressing their many similarities. Thanks to expanding knowledge of how emotions arise and are handled in different areas in the brain, recognition of distinctive features has become possible.

A system where emotions can be divided into either positive or negative carries a certain appeal. Happiness, love, and sympathy are examples of the former, while fear, anger, sadness and disgust represent the latter. Judging by body reactions, negative emotions may be perceived as more inductive of neurohormonal output, which may be why they have been more frequently implicated in adverse effects on the heart.

Emotions can also be simple or complex, pure or mixed, and primary or secondary. The way emotions are processed in the brain probably provides a basis for the most scientific classification. There is general consensus that perceptions and basic emotions are processed at a "lower level" in areas called the limbic system* including the amygdala, the cingulated gyrus and other ventral areas. Certain selectivity is observed, including predilection for fear in the amygdala and joy in the hypothalamus. But there seems to be no absolute exclusivity in the system. A certain type of sudden emotional outburst can theoretically overwhelm the lower level (limbic area) while simultaneously, the higher cortical levels (that require additional time) cannot deal with such outburst, consuming inputs and utilization of learned experience. There are enough reasons to suspect that if shocking enough, emotions of this nature can stun the heart muscle by the associated outpouring of stress hormones causing what we came to know as the "Broken Heart Syndrome". In the milder forms, transient manifestations occur including rapid heart beating, pale discoloration due to constriction of vascular beds, and occasionally fainting.

On the other hand, more sustained handling of traumatic situations and the more complex experiences, such as coping with the loss of a loved one, are processed at higher levels in the cortex of the brain,* cardinal among them is prefrontal cortex. The amygdala may still serve as the initial recipient of the stimulus before they conduct it to the higher cortical areas where a more elaborate and time consuming process takes place. This multifaceted process involves thoughts, memories and learning experiences that can eventually lead to adaptation. Failure of the assimilation process may result in ongoing struggle and inability to cope, which may lead to the Post-traumatic Stress Disorder as described by Horowitz and others. This course of events is by no means benign but likely to exert its harmful effects on the heart and the circulatory system over the long term. Sustained stress, also called unresolved stress, is currently acknowledged as a major risk factor for heart disease and hypertension. Reports have already surfaced revealing significantly higher incidence of heart attacks in patients who suffer from the post-traumatic Stress Disorder. A more detailed discussion of acute and chronic forms of heart disease secondary to emotional trauma is to follow.

How can a cardiologist, with limited experience in Neurology and Psychiatry, or other non-medically oriented individuals view emotions

---

* Limbic system: a complex of several structures also known as the intermediate brain. It includes the amygdala and hippocampus. The system governs emotions and behavior.
* Brain cortex: the outer layer of the brain consisting of "grey matter" made of neurons. The cortex plays a key role in memory, awareness, attention, language and thoughts.

from a global perspective? Recently, I have been fascinated by a comparison with colors. The basic colors of the light spectrum are compared with the basic emotions. Variable mixture of two colors creates new colors with still recognizable components of the original two. This can be compared with a second tier of emotions created by mergers that may include love, sympathy or pleasure.

As more colors enter into the mixture, and in a paralleled manner more emotions become involved adding to the 'complexity, a third or even higher tier results leading eventually to complex personality disorders and even aberrant behavior. This scheme allows me to plug in emotional phenomena or states of mind, and deranged behavior that cannot otherwise be placed in context. Examples are many, to name a few: love, hatred, frustration, revenge, selfishness, altruism, compassion, apathy, hope, paranoia, boredom, envy, and progressively into more complexity such as hysteria, aggression, obsession, sadism, masochism, criminality, etc.

CHAPTER FIVE

EMOTIONAL HEART DISEASE

"Hearts Tormented by Emotions"

THE CLINICAL SYNDROMES

The preceding four chapters address a general understanding of heart disease and where potential interactions with emotions may be operative. This will set the stage for the main discussion on the recently popularized link between emotions and heart disease. The following chapters will address the early recognition of heart disease in the absence of diseased arteries, and the subsequent mounting evidence pointing to a relationship with emotions and stress. Later, the clinical manifestations including currently well known emotionally related conditions will be discussed.

Can a Bump on the head cause a heart attack?

Acute Heart Attack After severe Emotional Shock Due to Head Trauma

Excruciating pain coupled with fear, especially if it is of a sudden onset, can serve as a stimulus for the outpouring of stress hormones adrenalin, noradrenalin and other reactive stress proteins, such as Neuropeptide Y and Serotonin. A **35-year-old man** who had no risk factors for heart disease was working in a factory when a metal bar fell and struck his head. He developed a "terrible" headache and was emotionally shocked by **surprise** and **fear.** Soon afterwards, he felt severe chest pain, dizziness, nausea, and diaphoresis. An electrocardiogram done in the emergency ambulance showed unequivocal signs of hyperacute heart attack involving the whole front wall of the heart. This almost certainly means total occlusion of the important left anterior descending coronary artery. This was documented by coronary angiography.

At the time, the standard practice did not include attempts to promptly re-open the artery in the heart catheterization laboratory and, due to severe head trauma, acute thrombolytic therapy with potent blood thinners, was considered as contraindicated for fear of inducing brain hemorrhage.

Nevertheless, the patient did well clinically with progressive improvement. Several days later a repeated coronary angiogram proved what we had suspected: a wide-open artery with some irregularity at the distal end, probably due to small clots. The evidence is strong in this case that emotional shock (with components of fear, surprise, pain, and frustration) served as a potent stimulus for instant release of stress hormones and other substances that caused severe spasm, totally blocking the coronary artery with clot formation and a heart attack.

Emotional stress stimulates the release of catecholamines and neurotransmitters so called stress hormones such as noradrenaline, adrenaline dopamine and serotonin; therefore, it is only logical to attribute any disturbances of heart function to their actions. A dual mechanism was suspected to explain neurotransmitters effects on the heart and vascular system. On the one hand these chemicals are capable of promoting frank spasm or increased vascular tone in coronary arteries and other arterial beds throughout the body. This can cause ischemia by reduced supply as opposed to that due to increased demand (see chapter 1). A combination of spasm and atherosclerotic obstruction is not uncommon and is highlighted by the syndrome of Prinzmetal angina. On the other hand, stress hormones exert a direct damaging effect on the myocardial muscle fibers even in the absence of arterial blockage. This effect on the muscle is due to direct toxic action, diffuse disease in small arteries running within the muscle and not normally visible on the angiogram, or both at the same time.

EMOTION-RELATED ANGINA - *"LOVE BITES"*
Angina due to Coronary Spasm

Traditionally, the anginal syndrome of typical chest pain occurring on activity and relieved by rest has been attributed to obstructive coronary artery disease. With the advent of coronary cineangiography by Mason Sones, this relationship was firmly established. This is particularly true if the pain is associated with abnormal electrocardiogram showing signs consistent with ischemia. These signs typically include horizontal depression of a line called ST segment and or the downward inversion of a normally upright wave called the T wave. Acute heart attacks, on the other hand, are heralded by similar chest pain, only more severe, that occurs mostly at rest—especially in the early morning hours, often accompanied by profuse diaphoresis (sweating) and occasionally nausea, vomiting, dizziness, or palpitations. Usually the symptoms are not abated by complete rest. The most objective test to separate angina from a heart attack is, again, the electrocardiogram. Today this can be done by the paramedics team in the home, on the field, or promptly upon arrival at the ER. This test shows, in the case of a heart attack, an elevation of the ST segment in contrast with the depression seen in simple angina. Naturally different measures described earlier in this book will have to be implemented should a heart attack be suspected. The paramedics Team would start by assuring stability of heart rhythm and administering certain intravenous medications if needed, or delivering what could be a life-saving electric shock if the heart is fibrillating. Potent pain medications are given in addition to nitroglycerine. Relief of pain is especially important since persistent pain leads to stress and anxiety which in turn results in further need for the already meager oxygen carrying blood. The ultimate intervention is done in the hospital by prompt transfer to the catheterization laboratory and an attempt to re-open the blocked artery. The sooner this can be accomplished the more complete the recovery would be. Indeed, the elapsed time between arrival to the ER and reestablishing blood flow in the affected artery is considered a major index of quality and preparedness of the hospital involved.

The first variance from this traditional scenario was observed by Prinzmetal in 1959. He described a fascinating syndrome in which the pain and the finding on electrocardiogram are identical to those of an acute heart attack. The only difference is that the complaint will subside either spontaneously or after the administration of nitroglycerine, therefore behaving like regular angina. Almost ten years following Prinzmetal account, the availability of coronary Cineangiography revealed most frequently the presence of severe narrowing of the coronary artery in contrast with the complete blockage found in a true heart attack. Transient total occlusion of the artery that reverses spontaneously or in response to nitroglycerine appears to provide the most plausible explanation. It was not until 1973, working with a team at George Washington University, that we documented that a subgroup of patients with Prinzmetal-like syndrome were found to have severe spasm of otherwise normal looking artery by angiography, a new ischemic phenomenon we called "A Variant of the Variant" which can readily explain Prinzmetal type angina. If spasm alone can block a fully patent artery, it can certainly do the same to an already severely narrowed but not totally blocked one. The concept of spasm-induced ischemia was greatly enhanced by this revelation.

Anginal SYNDROME X

Later that same year we published our article on variant angina, the cardiologists' community was puzzled by a review describing a large number of patients with typical angina associated with normal coronary arteriogram. A total of 200 patients were evaluated over 6 years. Over 50% of patients had changes on the electrocardiogram suggestive of ischemia. Exercise test was abnormal in only about 20% of patients consistent with non-exercise induced ischemia in the majority of patients. This provided further support to reduced blood supply as the cause of ischemia, which can be explained by coronary artery spasm. In patients with metabolic evidence of ischemia, women were 3 times more frequent than men. This syndrome, later referred to as syndrome X, was found to be relatively benign with more than half of the patients improving spontaneously without specific therapy for angina. Mortality over 6 years was comparable with the matching "normal" group from actuarial data. The authors proposed multi-factorial etiology of this syndrome that included psychosomatic factors, coronary artery spasm, and disease primarily affecting small vessels traversing the heart muscle.

Psychosomatic Angina

After our report on spasm-induced angina in otherwise normal looking coronary angiogram, we stayed on the lookout for clues on how spontaneous spasm can occur. We already had the experience— from our work and the work of others—that coronary arteries can occasionally undergo severe spasm in selected patients when they are inadvertently "irritated" mechanically by catheters or wires used during heart catheterization procedures. The fact that this is not observed in many patients suggests a special predisposition in some. Anecdotal observations suggested a special predilection for females and the right coronary artery in particular.

The tendency for coronary spasm can be evaluated in suspected cases by injection into the arteries of an ergotamine compound (Ergonovin) that can reproduce both anginal pain and angiographically evident spasm. The test introduced by Heupler has since been practically abandoned. Another vasoactive substance, acetylcholine—normally inductive of arterial dilatation, was found to paradoxically cause constriction in individuals predisposed for coronary spasm. Pharmacological testing as outlined above is rarely, if ever, used nowadays in clinical settings largely because we now accept that in a patient with non-obstructed coronary arteries, spasm is probably the only logical mechanism for ischemia at rest.

Special predilection in the female 'gender raises a serious question of whether women are more likely than men to develop coronary artery spasm, and also whether certain women are more predisposed than others?

Our team evaluated in a prospective manner nine consecutive patients who manifested typical angina with unmistakable signs of ischemia on the electrocardiogram and who were found to have normal coronary angiograms. All were women; this time we obtained detailed emotional and psychosocial profiles of all. Astonishing similarities were found between these women. Common features were almost uniformly observed including the following:

- All were between the ages of 45-65 and mostly postmenopausal.

- None volunteered information regarding her emotional or personal problems at the beginning of or during the detailed history-taking process.

- Almost all women broke into tears when asked if they were experiencing any current or recent traumatic emotional problem.

- In all, emotional trauma had a strong sexual content. Typically, self-esteem was lowered due to recent divorce, adultery, sexual neglect, and lack of fulfillment. In two of the women, there were sexual and drug abuse problems with young teenage children. None admitted to having been battered.

These findings clearly suggest that post-menopausal females who suffer from psycho-emotional problems with strong sexual content are primarily prone to coronary spasm with angina and even heart attacks.

It is not clear whether peri-menopausal women are more predisposed because of a biological hormonal imbalance, or simply since these types of problems tend to occur more frequently around this age. A combination of both seems likely. Nitroglycerine, tranquilizers, and spasm relieving medications such as the group of drugs called calcium-blocking agents all proved to be helpful. These medications given isolated or in combination were adequate to control anginal pain in these women. However, occasionally, professional psychotherapy was needed. Relapses were observed but remissions lasting one year or more were common. None of the patients developed features of definite myocardial infarction.

In summary these findings suggest that angina due to reduced blood supply to the heart in this group of women is probably the result of coronary artery spasm due to excessive release of stress hormones provoked by emotional conflicts. Widespread constriction of coronary arteries or frank spasm in certain areas can both explain this phenomenon. Moreover, patients known to have true atherosclerotic coronary artery disease may experience increasing frequency of pain episodes during periods of anxiety and stress. It seems that the threshold for pain in these patients is lowered by an increase in stress hormones.

"BROKEN HEARTS" CAN CAUSE HEART ATTACKS

Not only angina can occur or worsen due to emotional stress, but a real heart attack can also happen. In 1972 we reported one of the earliest, if not the first, demonstrations of acute heart attack due to spasm in the circumflex coronary artery. If coronary spasm can induce ischemia, then profound persistent spasm can certainly cause a full heart attack. The difference between the two conditions lies basically in the severity and duration of the spastic episode. However, with persistent spasm, other factors may enter into play. Among the most common and most serious is clot formation. This can be enhanced by stagnation of blood flow with subsequent activation of blood platelets and other clotting factors. Maseri advanced a "unifying hypothesis" that includes plaque rupture, increased sensitivity to stress hormones and clot formations that work in concert to occlude the artery completely and result in a heart attack. It is likely that spasm provoked by emotional stress works as the initial trigger in these cases.

Utilizing these basic principles, we explained our experience with another group of eight patients (6 women, 2 men) over a five year period who suffered acute heart attacks without any clear evidence of atherosclerotic disease. Coronary angiography was normal in 5 and showed severe spasm in 2 and spasm plus blood clot in 1. Psychosocial history was sought, and five patients out of the eight gave a history of typical chest pain occurring subsequent to heightened emotional activity. In two of these, heart attack occurred during the course of severe emotional experience. Seven of the eight patients admitted to having been suffering from ongoing mostly unvented emotional stress. Again, we have observed the higher frequency of this condition in women. One patient with severe diffuse spasm of the very important left anterior descending coronary artery had total failure of function in a large portion of the main pumping chamber (the left ventricle), typical to the condition we now know as "Apical Ballooning Syndrome" or "Tako-tsubo Stress Cardiomyopathy." These two "strange" names will be clarified later.

After reporting this paper I wrote a brief editorial in a local San Mateo newspaper under the title "Broken Hearts Can Cause Heart Attacks". This helped draw direct public attention to a potential risk of worsening heart function as a result of severe emotional stress.

Heart Attack Due To Amphetamine Abuse

Both heart attacks and heart muscle disease (cardiomyopathy) have been reported in association with amphetamine abuse. The drastic complication of this "recreational drug" can occur whether it was used via inhalation, oral route or intravenously. Like emotional stress, myocardial damage is thought to be mediated by catecholamines. Potential mechanisms include coronary artery vasospasm, direct catecholamines-induced myocardial damage, or an effect on blood platelets promoting their aggregation and subsequent formation of a clot that can block the flow of blood in a coronary artery and lead to a heart attack.

In 1994, I **reported a unique case of a 29 year-old woman** who was victim to a similar scenario. After initial evidence of injury in the lower (inferior) portion of the heart, her symptoms improved with intravenous administration of nitroglycerine, a potent coronary artery dilator. On the following day she developed chest pain again and the ECG reflected a similar but larger early heart attack, this time involving the front portion of her heart. She was immediately moved for urgent catheterization and coronary angiography. The latter revealed the presence of a filling defect in the artery most compatible with a clot. Despite the resulting damage, the patient survived, albeit with partially weakened heart.

The importance of cases like these is that they seem to verify the dual mechanisms of amphetamine-induced heart damage. This first implies spasm induced by catecholamines stress hormones and the second, clot formation that continues to block the artery after the spasm has resolved.

Action of amphetamine on coronary arteries resulting in heart attacks cannot fully explain direct heart muscle damage and failure seen in many abusers of this drug. Heart damage cannot be simply explained by blockage of a large artery; it is rather diffuse and globally weakens the heart over an extended period of time. Widespread constriction of the whole network system of small arteries directly supplying the heart muscle will have to be implicated. It has also been postulated that there is a direct damaging effect on the muscle itself, unrelated to the vascular system. A similar mechanism is also suspected in heart muscle damage associated with cocaine addiction. Furthermore heart muscle damage can occur in association with pheochromocytoma* a tumor that grows on the adrenal gland located on top of each kidney. The normal levels of stress hormone secretion from this gland are markedly higher, which can result in widespread heart muscle damage, similar to that seen in amphetamine and cocaine abuse.

A recent scientific statement from The American Heart Association on cocaine-associated chest pain and myocardial infarction is of special interest. The statement requests that when treating a patient with chest pain who has no obvious risks of heart disease, doctors should ask if the patient has used cocaine. Cocaine use is now established as a possible cause of angina as well as heart attacks.

"THE STRAW THAT BROKE THE CAMEL'S BACK"

This is the case of a 75 year-old man who suffered chest pain within a few minutes after hearing of the death of a dearly beloved nephew. The pain propagated into a major heart attack with full electrocardiographic features. Expeditious intervention with coronary artery angiogram upon arriving in the hospital revealed extensive narrowing of all major arteries. The culprit artery was re-canalized and a coronary stent was deployed to keep it open. All the features of a heart attack were dramatically reversed, with subsequent stable hospital course and safe discharge.

This case is not unique and suggests that spasm superimposed on top of real arterial disease may provide the "straw that broke the camel's back." Just consider how many emotional "straws" there are on any given day of our modern lives that can break the "back" of a heart al-

---

* Pheochromocytoma: a tumor that grows on the adrenal glands and secretes abnormally high amounts of adrenaline and noradrenaline that result in elevated blood pressure as well as heart muscle damage.

ready burdened by diseased arteries and commonly high blood pressure as well. Think of the variety of emotions with "negative" contents that can happen over the course of a week—such as fear, frustration, sadness, envy, surprise, disgust, shame, guilt, loneliness, and even boredom, to name a few. Vulnerability varies between individuals, and unfortunately it is usually recognized only after the event. With no "vaccine" or "magic bullet" currently available against potential adverse effects of emotions (and none clearly on the horizon), this problem is likely to remain for the foreseeable future. Moreover, if the lives of ordinary people continue to increase in complexity with ever more challenges and frustrations, the extent of medical and psychosocial repercussions is expected to steadily grow.

One of the widespread daily activities that frequently constitute a source of stress and frustration is **driving to work** The need to rush to work can sometimes result in heightened levels of stress, anxiety, and frustration. We have recently encountered the following case and we have already published a similar one to illustrate the potentially serious cardiac events associated with traffic related stress.

Can a Traffic Jam cause a Heart Attack?

Heart Attack and Loss Of Consciousness In The Midst of Traffic-Related Anxiety and Frustration

Rushing to get to work on time, Alex a **42 year-old man** caught in stalled traffic was feeling, in his own words, "very nervous and frustrated." He started feeling an oppressive pain in the front of his chest. Soon after, he felt dizzy but managed to pull his car to the emergency lane before completely losing consciousness. Upon arrival of the paramedics, he was awake but continuing to suffer from the same symptoms. Localized myocardial infarction within the wall of the pumping chamber (not traversing the thickness of the wall) was diagnosed in the emergency room by the markedly elevated Troponin—a highly sensitive and specific marker of heart muscle damage—as well as electrocardiographic changes indicating an interruption of blood supply to the heart. Urgent cardiac catheterization revealed a less than critical narrowing in a large right coronary artery with a normal left system. The most reasonable hypothesis was that the affected artery became totally blocked at the time. This compromised the supply of blood to the electrical conduction system of the heart, causing either a heart standstill or a very slow heart rate. This in turn triggered the loss of consciousness. What can explain this? Stress related spasm and total occlusion for a period of time long enough to cause a small heart attack before spontaneous resolution of the spasm and therefore the blockage.

In view of the tendency of this moderate (60%) lesion to undergo spasm in reaction to emotional stress, we decided to proceed with intervention and deployment of a coronary stent. Ordinarily we do not resort to stent insertion in lesions of this moderate severity. However, we believe that if such a lesion is proven to be capable of causing a life threatening event, it is safer to treat it preventively with a stent. The message from this case is that emotional reactions that appear on the surface to be trivial or even "normal" during our daily life may not be truly so. Just think of the potential sources of aggravations we encounter everyday, of which traffic stress is only one example. Real heart damage is particularly likely to occur in individuals made vulnerable by a special disposition for coronary artery spasm.

So far we have learned how coronary artery spasm induced by emotional stress can cause a heart attack. Such cases probably represent a small portion of all heart attack cases. The importance of the concept of emotionally related spasm goes beyond the numbers. Just consider this: if spasm can cause heart attacks in people with apparently normal coronary arteries, it can certainly do damage to those with diseased ones. In fact, even less potent emotional stress is needed to complete the blockage of an already narrowed artery. This is even more probable if the pre-existing narrowing is severe. Such a concept, if proven, can have far-reaching implications by providing an explanation for why a heart attack can rapidly develop in individuals who had previously recognized stable coronary disease. Since sudden emotional episodes can occur consciously or in the subconscious as well as in connection with dreams, their role in triggering acute cardiac events is quite significant. While emotional crisis can trigger a classic heart attack, they can also cause serious or potentially fatal heart rhythm disorders in lieu of a full-fledged heart attack. Let us review the case of an older man who experienced events that follow the above logic.

CHAPTER SIX

HEART MUSCLE FAILURE DUE TO EMOTIONAL STRESS

(THE BROKEN HEART SYNDROME)

"BROKEN HEART" After the Loss of a Young Granddaughter

Emily at 80 years old was in excellent health. All of a sudden she started to have breathing difficulty, (dyspnea) and congestion in her lungs (increased fluid in the lungs). These symptoms followed the death of her six year-old granddaughter, who she described as her only reason to "stay alive". Her granddaughter died of acute leukemia, an almost universally and usually rapidly fatal form of blood cancer. The electrocardiogram showed nonspecific changes. An echocardiogram confirmed severe reduction of heart function mainly the apical area and adjacent portions of the heart muscle. The normal value of ejection fraction of over 55% was less than 20%. Significant but transient improvement followed the intravenous infusion of Dobutamine a heart function stimulating substance. Within one week, the function of the heart muscle was back to near normal range. A noninvasive nuclear test for coronary artery disease came out normal. The Dobutamine infusion test also showed no evidence of a persistent problem. Sorrow and grief will never depart the soul of this elderly woman, yet her heart muscle has learned how to adjust.

Stunning Of Heart Function Due To Emotional Shock

The recent description of this syndrome in medical literature has captured appreciable interest in the medical community and the public at large. The dramatic deterioration of heart function after an emotional shock such as the sudden loss of a loved one is the hallmark of this increasingly recognized condition. Vascular collapse can occur and even death has been reported. A classical case is associated with symptoms of breathing difficulty and discomfort in the chest, serious concern arises after detecting abnormalities on the electrocardiogram. However, it is mostly after the discovery on the echocardiogram of markedly reduced mechanical function of a large area of the left ventricle that the concern really heightens. Nearly complete loss of function typically involving the apical portion is observed. This latter finding can lead to suspicion of a traditional heart attack. Adding to the confusion, the levels in the blood of cardiac enzymes related to heart damage such as Creatinine Phosphokinase and Troponin may be elevated. Nevertheless, the classical pattern of acute myocardial infarction is usually lacking, and most importantly recovery of heart muscle function is the rule in most cases. This striking stunning of function carries the imprints of a catecholamine surge, and its initial levels are found to be markedly increased. Before going into more details, I would like to present two illustrative cases of this syndrome that we have recently encountered.

CAN PAIN AND FEAR STUN THE HEART?

Jennifer, a 72 year-old woman with lung cancer was found to have pericardial effusion (fluid accumulation inside the pericardial sac surrounding the heart) that was suspected of causing compression on the heart, a complication medically called Tamponade. Due to the fear of dire consequences and the need to analyze the fluid, a procedure called "pericardiocentesis" was advised, whereby the fluid is removed using a long needle advanced under local anesthesia. Being aware of the serious nature of her medical condition, along with the mounting pain, apprehension and fear, the patient did not tolerate the procedure well. She became nervous and extremely "stressed out". At this point her heart function, as observed by echocardiography monitor, became extremely poor, dropping from a normal ejection fraction value of 60% to less than 15%. The patient suffered from symptoms of heart failure and required treatment. Eventually left ventricular function recovered as seen by a follow up echo test. The fear of a painful and potentially risky medical procedure has also been observed to cause acute and transient severe heart muscle stunning.

SCARED OF AN OPERATION!
FEAR AND APPREHENSION PRIOR TO
SURGICAL PROCEDURE

Jackie, a **65-year old woman** was quite apprehensive and frightened prior to having a scheduled operation to repair a torn rotator cuff in her shoulder. She was reassured by a cardiology consultant that her examination, ECG, and Echocardiogram were all normal. Her fear peaked while she was on the operative table being prepared for induction of anesthesia. Suddenly she suffered cardiac arrest with marked drop in her blood pressure and very slow heart rate of less than 20 beats per minute. She became unresponsive. Heart resuscitation measures were fully and promptly implemented and she was intubated and placed on a ventilator. Follow up echocardiogram in the intensive care unit showed her left heart function was at fifteen percent with complete lack of function at the apex and surrounding area giving the typical appearance frequently encountered in stress cardiomyopathy and describes as apical ballooning. Within five days the patient achieved full clinical recovery including the return of her heart function to the normal level of over sixty percent.

Increased attention to this condition has led to greater awareness and recognition of the scope of its severity and apparent relationship to acute emotional stress. Milder cases are probably common but, due to lack of symptoms, they are likely to go undiscovered. Therefore, the actual prevalence is not yet determined. The mere existence of this medical condition independently from other known forms of heart disease illustrates the need to reach a full understanding of all its aspects. This includes predisposition, coexistence with other disease states, triggering events, as well as the potential for preventive and therapeutic measures. The frequently stunned area of the ventricle does not clearly match with the distribution of one large coronary artery suggesting that large artery spasm is not the usual mechanism. More likely, stress hormones exert their effects on smaller arteries traversing the thickness of the heart muscle. Furthermore, it is possible that more protracted cases can develop leading to progressive and potentially irreversible damage to the heart muscle. If so, can unrelenting stress lead to chronic heart muscle disease (cardiomyopathy)? Can the process of a vicious cycle of remodeling* be operative and eventually lead to progressively worsening

---

* Remodeling of the heart describes progressive enlargement in the chamber with gradually worsening function after a severe damage in a sizeable area of the pumping chamber (left ventricle).

function? From what we know now, recovery is the rule; therefore, medications are given basically to alleviate troubling symptoms. Finally, is there a role in the management for psychotherapy? Can future research succeed in identifying susceptible individuals? The statistical evidence at present seems to indicate that the condition is mainly seen in older women.

In summary emotional heart disease, whether related to coronary arterial spasm or to stunning of the heart muscle, is much more common in women. Answers to the questions raised above remain, to a large extent, speculative. It is hoped that the increased interest in this subject will allow researchers to uncover the mysteries of emotional heart disease. This will undoubtedly lead to an improvement in the prevention and in the treatment.

CHAPTER SEVEN

EXPANSIVE RECOGNITION OF EMOTIONAL HEART DISEASE

"An Open Pandora's Box"

Recognition of emotional heart disease, in particular the understanding of the mediators involved in its production, has greatly expanded over the past two decades. Today it is mainly accepted that Catecholamine's onslaught on the heart targets the large coronary arteries as well as their branching tree of small vessels, traversing the thickness of the heart muscle. In addition, a direct toxic effect on the cardiac muscle itself is also likely. Catecholamines work in concert with other stress compounds such as Serotonin and Y. Peptide. Endothelial dysfunction* creates more harmful effects by producing endothelin—an artery-constricting substance—and preventing the production of helpful artery-dilating substances, such as Prostacycline and Nitric Oxide. Constriction of coronary arteries may ensue; this can be focal, involving a short segment or widespread and therefore more threatening. This concept has lead to a "revival" of the interest in coronary spasm, after having been shelved for decades since it was proposed by Osler. As noted earlier, the advent of coronary Cineangiography helped to confirm its role. Inciting factors include exposure to cold, mechanical irritation by catheters, and certain drugs such as Ergotamine, a compound used for the treatment of migraine headache attacks. Spontaneous spasm of angiographically normal-looking arteries has been demonstrated by our team, as well as by others.

Subsequent case reports and large clinical studies and investigations continued to emerge in the literature pioneered by Maseri, Chierchia, Yasue, Heupler, and others. The search for the elusive trigger or triggers of coronary events including unstable angina, heart attacks and sudden death, has been greatly enhanced by the recognition of the potential role of coronary spasm.

---

* endothelial dysfunction: disruption of the highly protective layer of cells lining the inside of an artery.

In a comprehensive recent review of factors that can trigger acute cardiovascular events, Toffler and Muller outlined all proven causes. Their review was loaded with inferences to emotional and emotionally related factors, with emphasis on psychosocial disturbances, stress, and emotional enrage. The direct relation to heightened anger, anxiety, and fear is of special prominence. Increased mortality was also observed in widowers and during disasters afflicting mass populations. In this chapter I will discuss stressful conditions that are proven or highly suspected of inducing heart disease, either in acute dramatic fashion or insidiously over an extended period. I will also address variable knowledge on the natural history in a large number of patients as new information on this subject has started to emerge.

MANY NAMES, SAME DISEASE EMOTIONAL ACUTE HEART STUNNING :
A.k.a. Stress Cardiomyopathy "Tako-tsubo Cardiomyopathy," "Apical Ballooning Syndrome," or "Broken Heart Syndrome"

Reported independently within the last decade, all these terms have probably described the same condition of acute—usually reversible—left ventricular apical stunning secondary to sudden emotional stress. The similarities were obviously pointing essentially to a single disease entity. Its relationship with emotional outbursts is now uniformly recognized. The suspicion that catecholamines are the mediators was strongly supported by the remarkable finding by Wittstein et al of excessively elevated levels exceeding by several times those found in true myocardial infarction, and up to 34 times the normal values. In a little over a week these values declined to less than one half of their peaks. While other factors cannot be excluded these findings point to a strong link between emotional shock, onslaught of stress hormones, and myocardial stunning. Death of a loved one was the trigger in about one half of the patients. Other causes centered mostly around acute fear or apprehension. In most reported cases of this syndrome, mild elevation of cardiac enzymes was observed, and subtle electrocardiographic changes indicative of ischemia were also common.

The parallel syndrome described in Japan is named "Tako-tsubo Cardiomyopathy," due to the similarity between the heart configuration and that of a fishing instrument used to trap octopus. While not initially attributed to emotional stress, evidence has since pointed heavily in favor of this relationship. The Tako-tsubo configuration and ventricular stunning were first described by Dote et al in 1991. Several reportings also appeared later in Japanese literature, raising suspicion that the Japanese people are more prone to this condition. However, in 2005, Scott et al reported a nearly identical condition in a prospective clinical study of 22 American, non-Japanese females, mostly over the age of 50 years. This and other experiences published later from different nations in variable ethnic populations have all but dispelled the notion of a special selection for the Japanese.

Heart Failure due to Pregnancy; Postpartum Cardiomyopathy*

This is an infrequently encountered form of heart stunning. This disease is characterized by new enlargement of the heart in late pregnancy and after delivery that can result in heart failure. The cause is unknown but the condition typically worsens with subsequent pregnancies. The similarities with stress cardiomyopathy are noticeable. These include rapid development and tendency for spontaneous improvement. Here again, probable relation to hormonal factors and stress is likely.

MYOCARDIAL STUNNING AND HEART ATTACKS DURING NATURAL DISASTERS

The incidence of heart attacks is reportedly increased during natural disasters. Catastrophic events of sudden and unexpected onset associated with rapid devastation and loss of human life are particularly implicated. The trigger mechanism probably involves a sudden and powerful mix of emotions including fear, surprise, and frustration. The total unpredictability of earthquakes and their inflicted devastation at a lightening speed make them the more likely of all major disasters to trigger heart attacks and emotional stunning of the heart. Indeed, frequent medical reports of retrospective analysis have confirmed this suspicion. Watanabe et al evaluated the frequency of cardiac events during one week following major earthquake activity in Niigata, Japan and

---

* Postpartum cardiomyopathy is not a fully understood condition. It affects women in late pregnancy and after delivery. Depending on severity and recurrence with subsequent pregnancies, severe failure may ensue occasionally requiring heart transplantation

found a marked increase in heart attacks and sudden death. The number of cases of Tako-tsubo cardiomyopathy, a primarily emotion-related condition, increased twenty five fold during the four weeks following the earthquakes by comparison with the same 4 week periods a year and 2 years before. Similar increase was also observed during the 1994 Northridge earthquake in Los Angeles, California and the Athens earthquake in 1982. Interestingly, similar increases were also found in other types of catastrophic events including the Iraqi missile attacks on Israel in 1991, and the terrorist attack on the world trade center in 2001. Events inductive of heightened emotional frustration without real tragedies can also be associated with increased cases of heart attacks. An example is the 1996 European football final when Holland lost very narrowly to France. An increase in cases of heart attacks and strokes was reported this time in Dutch males. Furthermore, sudden death during sex, called by the French "La mort douce", or "sweet death," was found to be much more frequent in adulterous sex, presumably as a result of fear and/or guilt. In conclusion, not only personal and private acute stress can lead to heart attack or stunning, but so can mass emotional shocks spreading fear, helplessness, disappointment or perceived "disaster".

ACUTE STROKES CAN ALSO LEAD TO STUNNING OF THE HEART

Brain injury from acute strokes due to blood clots or cerebral hemorrhage may be associated with sudden and occasionally severe heart failure. When a **brain aneurysm*** bursts, causing hemorrhage in the subarachnoid space, changes on the electrocardiogram suggestive of heart muscle injury are frequently observed. Heart muscle enzyme levels in the blood may also rise. Heart failure not unlike that seen during emotional heart stunning may ensue and result in excessive fluid congestion in both lungs. A condition medically named **"Neurogenic Pulmonary Edema"**—a surge in stress hormones and increased blood pressure levels—are implicated. Changes in endothelial function of small vessels within the lungs can render them incompetent, which leads to leakage of fluid into lung tissue, aggravating pulmonary edema.

---

* Brain aneurysm is a bulging sac out of a brain artery. It may occasionally rupture due to high blood pressure or gradual expansion, causing frequently large hemorrhage within the brain.

Direct catecholamines' mediated injury of lungs tissue has also been suspected.

Neurogenic heart stunning as the case in emotional stunning is usually reversible. In the setting of dangerous cerebral accidents, the prognosis is not as good and death may result from the extensive brain injury itself. The following is case presentation that further supports the link between the brain and heart stunning.

HEART ATTACK AT THE ONSET OF MULTIPLE SCLEROSIS
From the brain to the heart

The onset of multiple sclerosis a serious central nervous disease of unclear cause can be very subtle or on the contrary quite dramatic with new visual defects.

Norma, a 21 year-old female was admitted with chest pain and found to have typical features of an acute heart attack, including findings on the electrocardiogram and elevation of the levels of heart enzymes in the blood. She had complained for several days of visual changes, headache, and dizziness. Prompt evaluation by heart catheterization revealed severe suppression of heart function to less than 40% and normal coronary arteries. She was placed on medications and general intensive care management. Later, and consistent with stress cardiomyopathy, heart function was nearly fully recovered within one week. Despite this, we were still apprehensive about her brain symptoms.

Specialized studies in the immunology laboratory and Magnetic Resonance Imaging (MRI) of the brain confirmed the diagnosis of new onset of multiple sclerosis. The patient was started on the appropriate treatment. Two months later, a follow-up ECG and Echocardiogram were normal. This case supports the existence of a brain-heart connection most probably mediated by neurohormonal and sympathetic nerve discharge. This can result in heart suppression typical of the "Broken Heart Syndrome".

The Brain-Heart Axis:

Interaction between the heart and the brain has been suspected for many years. Emotional outburst—including rage, marked anxiety and occasionally sexual activity—are commonly associated with angina pain, rapid heart rate and high blood pressure. Stage fright or pre-examination nervousness are other examples. This mutual exchange between the heart and the brain can work at times in the other direction. Depression is fairly common after heart attacks. The level of depression usually correlates well with the severity of heart dysfunction as assessed clinically or by measurement of certain parameters of heart function.

An increasing number of cases are being reported that illustrate the importance of the brain-heart axis. Emotional factors, including depression, are the most prominent examples. This is especially operative in older overweight women, and to a much smaller extent in men. Depression has a major impact on the central nervous system. Stress hormones and behavioral patterns are altered so as to exert a more adverse influence on heart function. The impact of organic brain disease on the heart is probably still underestimated. As noted earlier, hemorrhage within the brain has been reported to cause profound suppressive effect on heart function. Other brain conditions especially depression can, hypothetically, induce a similar effect.

POST-TRAUMATIC STRESS DISORDER (PTSD) & THE HEART

PTSD is a protracted emotional condition that follows a major frightening experience, such as battlefield stress, rape, or other life-threatening experiences. Recent studies revealed that affected individuals are more prone to suffer from heart attacks later in life than the general population. This found relationship tends to support an association between chronic stress of a profound nature and heart disease, heart attacks in particular. Unlike acute emotional stress, which rapidly stuns the heart, chronic stress of this nature may exert its harm by predisposing for (namely atherosclerotic) coronary artery disease. Traditional treatment for coronary artery disease is usually needed. It is still important to recognize the emotional root of the condition and the frequent need for adjunct psychotherapy.

DEPRESSION CAN ALSO DEPRESSES THE HEART! "LOVE BIRDS"

Derek an 85 year-old man lost his 77 year old wife two months before he was admitted to the hospital with chest pain and breathless-ness, including other signs of heart failure. In addition, he became confused and, when awake and alert, he cried like a child. His daughter explained how close her parents had been.

Tests for his heart arteries were surprisingly normal at his advanced age. His daughter temporally suspended her professional work and fully dedicated her time to provide him with compassionate care. After one week in the hospital his heart failure symptoms as well as depression were progressively improving. In addition he regained much of his mental alertness and orientation. Despite the gravity of emotional heart disease in this elderly man, treatment was successful, thanks to psychosocial attention, physical therapy, medications, and, of course, time.

Several studies have found increased mortality from cardiovascular disease among depressed patients. Depression may start after a heart attack, usually indicating a worse prognosis. In depressed patients immediately after myocardial infarction, mortality rate was found to be 33 times higher than in non-depressed patients. Since many depressed individuals also smoke cigarettes, recent studies controlled for smoking were done and also showed an emerging direct relationship between depression and cardiovascular events. The proposed mechanism, again, points to stress hormones and the autonomous nervous system imbalance, as well as activation of the clotting factors called platelets, in patients suffering from depression.

A.J. Fagring et al published their experience from Sweden: they compared 127 men and 104 women with unexplained chest pain to a matched reference group without chest pain. They found that patients were more likely to be immigrants, had more symptoms of depression, anxiety and more perceived stress at work. This further illustrates the relationship between psychological factors and chest pain.

TROUBLED RELATIONSHIPS & HEART DISEASE

Strife through any relationship, marriage in particular, can lead to higher incidence of heart disease. Regardless of the type and nature of relationships, the quality seems to be what matters. Those engaged in the worst quality relationships are 34 times more likely to suffer from heart attacks and other forms of heart disease or sudden death. De Vogli, the lead researcher of a study at the University College of London that evaluated negative relationship in a large number of British civil servants, suspects that chronic stress is most probably responsible for this. A quest for biological evidence of stress in this group yielded the discovery of elevated levels of stress hormones and possibly an inflammatory process incited by stress. Treatment of negative relationships is another complex matter. First, there is no concrete proof that ending a negative relationship will provide effective prevention or healing. Furthermore, ending a relationship may prove not only to be ineffective, but may on occasion be counterproductive. Being unmarried or a loner was also shown to be hazardous to the heart and general health. By moving in the direction of a positive relationship, marriage counseling—if successful may help prevent or mend a broken heart.

FEAR AND THE HEART

Of the primal emotions, fear appears to be the most powerful. Fear ignites an intense brain process centered predominantly in the amygdala. The subsequent reaction in the body can be so profound rendering the individual literally "frozen". The surge of stress hormones can cause crushing chest pain not unlike that experienced during the course of a heart attack. Fear serves as warning sign that promotes the enlisting of body defenses to confront the impending danger. Intense fear, especially when of sudden onset and rapid development, can bring about harmful effects on the heart muscle, heart rate, and blood pressure. Coping with fear as some researchers have found is largely the product of a chemical reaction within the amygdala.

WHAT ABOUT ANGER?

Among negative emotion, anger ranks high when it comes to the direct harmful effects on the heart. In vulnerable individuals, anger, just like fear, can propagate rapidly into a "dangerous" zone in the form of a "fit" or outrage. Sudden weakening of the heart or coronary artery spasm is not unlikely to happen and can be especially armful to a predisposed and already diseased heart. If sudden collapse ensues, certain life-threatening arrhythmia can develop. Most recently, researchers from Yale University described a unique expression on the ECG, which can be a red flag warning of an impending problem. In some individuals, this "anger spike" may warrant in certain unstable patients surgical insertion of an automatic heart defibrillator.

NATURAL HISTORY IS UNPREDICTABLE

The natural history of stress cardiomyopathy remains only partially understood. Sharkey and Associates found in a large series that the future is not exactly predictable. Staying on guard is essential with regular follow up and testing. They also found an expanded list of potential causes that includes seemingly simple stress such as getting lost while driving at night, death of a pet, sense of loss after retirement, and sad or even happy anniversaries.

WOMEN ARE MORE VULNERABLE:

What seems to be emerging is a very striking predilection for women, in particular during their menopause or post-menopausal years. Of interest is the fact that our experience with spasm-related angina (vasospastic angina), published in 1983, also pointed to selectivity for middle-aged women suffering from intense unvented and unresolved emotional stress. Even though the two syndromes of vasospastic angina and myocardial stunning are not truly identical with one characterized by loss of mechanical function while the other is manifested by chest pain, a common mechanism may be operative in both. Large and rapid outpouring of stress hormones in addition to causing chest pain, can overwhelm and effectively paralyze a large portion of the heart muscle. In contrast, ongoing unresolved long-term emotional stress can be expected to cause a less dramatic and intermittent rise in stress hormones causing arterial spasm and therefore episodes of anginal pain. The difference may, therefore, lie in the volume and the duration of catecholamines release.

The real cause behind women's susceptibility to this syndrome still evades definitive explanation. The several theories advanced in order to answer this question seem to all be relevant, suggesting that they may be acting in concert. Sex hormone imbalance at this age may be of central importance. Emotional, social, and psychological factors undoubtedly enter into this interplay; women are thought to be more sensitive to emotional stress and more vulnerable to its harmful effects.

Furthermore sex hormones are known to have an appreciable impact on endothelial function and vascular reactivity in addition to interaction with the neurohormonal system, The reason for selective involvement of the apical area of the heart causing "apical ballooning" is not yet clear. The fact that outflow tract of the heart is smaller in women than in their male counterparts is believed by some to play a role.

Despite the lack of clear single explanation for why women are more prone for stress cardiomyopathy, the evidence is overwhelmingly in favor of this observation. A multi-factorial theory suggests that the factors mentioned earlier and yet other unknown ones may be acting together.

In conclusion, severe stress, the female gender and outpouring of endogenous catecholamines constitute the main features of this acute heart illness.

CAN SOME STRESS BE GOOD FOR US?

You can only find a handful of informed people who claim that a stress filled life is good for your brain, heart, and other organs. However, let us not forget that stress hormones, including adrenaline and cortisol, are released from our own adrenal glands as part of a defense strategy by our own specialized brain centers. The purpose is to help us survive. A check and balance system exists and is concerned with controlling the situation. When overwhelmed by an emotional reaction, an unchecked flood of hormones and neurotransmitters inflicts damage on the heart, amongst other organs.

What about a low, constant dose of stress? Like the kinds encountered in many driven and highly motivated individuals: students struggling through college examinations, young couples coping with job or unemployment pressures while striving to secure a home and raise children in today's challenging environments. Uncertainties stemming from different sources—including financial downturns, illness, and natural disasters—can also generate a level of ongoing stress.

Stress is intrinsic to every active lifestyle. The pressure to maintain growth and sustain lifestyle is often extremely demanding. Clearly not all stressed" people are overtly being harmed by stress, although they may remain constantly vulnerable and prone to nervous breakdowns and/or chronic depression. A small dose of stress helps many individuals to enhance memory and to balance otherwise labile emotions. "Reasonably tamed" stress can also help prevent excessive self-focused behavior and, therefore, strengthens resilience. Last but not least, controlled stress can sound the alarm and awaken self-defenses to face any impending danger. Ideally, we should learn how to control our stress and redirect its positive forces to our benefit.

CHAPTER EIGHT

MANAGEMENT OF EMOTIONAL HEART DISEASE

"How can you mend a broken heart?"

For the management of a newly recognized medical illness to be effective, it should be based on the full identification of this illness and knowledge of its mechanisms and natural course. While much is yet to be learned about Emotional Heart Disease, we seem to have amassed a great deal of information and we have made significant progress in the understanding of this condition. Despite this, treatment still targets the alleviation of symptoms, supporting the heart, and containing or preventing potential complications. A reasonably non-aggressive approach avoiding drugs and interventions—with their inevitable side affects and inherent risks—seems to be justified.

However, two exceptions should not be overlooked. The first is a potential for early complications, including heart rhythm disorders, heart failure, and cardiogenic shock. While rare, their impacts can be very serious, and their management may require complex therapeutic measures. This may include intravenous infusion of a variety of heart supporting drugs, mechanical respirators, or electronic pacemakers. Occasionally, more invasive intervention may be needed, such as the insertion of an assist device called Intra Aortic Balloon Pump (IABP), a system that offers a major helping hand to a struggling heart. Sudden death from shock or arrhythmia can occur. Once stability prevails, the outcome will likely be favorable. If recovery of myocardial stunning proves to be sluggish and uncertain, drugs usually used for treatment of traditional cardiomyopathy and for heart failure may be utilized, including the classes of beta-blockers, nitrate, ACE inhibitors, and, diuretics.

Occasionally more dramatic procedures may be required; if a weakened muscular structure—called the papillary muscle—fails to hold the leaflets of the mitral valve, a life-threatening leak to the left upper chamber may ensue. Early intervention with medications, IABP, or surgical repair of the damaged valve may be needed as lifesaving measures.

The second exception, unlike the first, is not well understood. It is unclear at present how many patients or what type of patients are not likely to achieve a full recovery and, instead, continue to run a protracted course that eventually leads to chronic cardiomyopathy and heart failure. Treatment at this stage should be tailored to the severity of the disease and the patient's level of discomfort. Until more reliable data is available, continuation of supportive medical treatment is the rule. However, as early signs of failure appear, a step-up approach should be followed starting with special "biventricular" pacemakers that synchronize the actions of both ventricles by electrical stimulation. Implantable defibrillators may also be utilized if life-threatening arrhythmias occur. The need for heart transplantation has not been reported, but may have to be considered if nothing else is working.

The overall mortality of acute stress-induced cardiomyopathy is estimated to be about 1 to 3 %. Let us now briefly address the selective treatment of each of the previously discussed clinical syndromes.

TREATMENT OF SPECIFIC SYNDROMES
Vasospartic angina with normal coronary angiogram

A strong association between this syndrome and the female gender is quite evident, especially in the middle age and post-menopausal years. Frank spasm in large coronary arteries or diffuse constriction in the larger pool of smaller vessels are usually implicated. It may be useful to obtain a basic psychological profile to help guide the treatment. Certain tranquilizers or antidepressants are helpful in some patients. For combating coronary spasm, nitrates and calcium channel blockers are the mainstream of pharmacological therapy, usually reserved for symptomatic patients. Beta-blockers, on the other hand, can be counterproductive in large artery spasm. The overall prognosis is favorable; the majority of patients exhibit gradual improvement without specific therapy.

EMOTIONAL AND STRESS-INDUCED HEART ATTACKS

Despite presentation at times with full traditional acute myocardial infarction, the overall prognosis of this condition is also good. Segmental left ventricular dysfunction may be transient and post-infarction chest pain is usually controllable with traditional medications.

Echocardiography should be utilized to assess left ventricular function and to identify the occasional development of ventricular aneurysm or thrombus formation.* More medical treatment, including blood thinners (anticoagulants) may be indicated in these cases.

EMOTIONALLY TRIGGERED ACUTE MYOCARDIAL INFARCTION WITH UNDERLYING SEVERE CORONARY ARTERY DISEASE

Emotional trauma and catecholamines over-shoot are implicated in triggering the onset of acute MI in patients who have been considered until then to be stable. The infarction itself should be treated emergently—including, if appropriate, prompt mechanical (angioplasty) re-canalization of the blocked artery, followed by treatment with beta-blockers, and antiplatelets or anticoagulants. Treatment directed to the emotional trigger may be needed as adjunct therapy. A significant number of these patients may require coronary artery bypass surgery.

ACUTE EMOTIONAL MYOCARDIAL STUNNING

As discussed earlier in this chapter, most patients surpass the injury and proceed to full recovery within two weeks. Exceptions to this benign course include early cardiogenic shock, serious arrhythmia, mitral valve insufficiency, and thrombus formation. Late complications are not well evaluated, but conversion into a chronic phase of cardiomyopathy may occur. The treatment will be the same as in non-stress related cardiomyopathy.

WHAT ABOUT PREVENTION?

Identification of individuals at risk is the cornerstone to designing a plan for prevention. When dealing with emotional heart disease, a few trends are emerging that can narrow the scope of the vulnerable population. First, the condition afflicts primarily the female gender, ex-

---

* Ventricular aneurysm is an expansion of the damaged area of the wall of the pumping chamber during muscle contraction into the opposite direction. It occasionally harbors a blood clot that can separate and may cause a stroke.

cluding nearly one half of the population. Second, most afflicted women are over the age of fifty, allowing more concentration on the older segment of the population. Third, some women leave the impression on their primary care doctors as being especially "hyper sensitive" and quite reactive emotionally. Physicians may be able to acquire the skills to suspect potential candidates for emotional heart problems. Fourth, associated conditions indicative of active stress hormones response, such as inappropriate increase in heart rate, labile hypertension, and low threshold for being "startled" may help raise the index of suspicion. Fifth, patients with other "vascular phenomenon," such as migraine headaches and vasculitis, may be more susceptible. Sixth, the index of suspicion should be raised during major catastrophic events, natural disasters, wartime, economic downturns and political and psychosocial upheavals. When a patient fits into a suspected high-risk group, more credibility should be given to his complaints, especially those of chest pain, shortness of breath, and palpitations. Early attention followed by screening diagnostic cardiac workup is recommended. It is likely that starting treatment at an early stage may reduce the intensity of the condition and even avert worsening of coronary spasm and heart mechanical function. Potentially helpful medications may include sedatives, beta-adrenergic blocking agents, calcium-channels blocking nitrates, and antihypertensive drugs. Psychiatric evaluation may prove to be more effective if started early.

IS IT HELPFUL OR EVEN ETHICAL TO MANIPULATE EMOTIONS?

Emotions and stress are tightly interrelated. They can in concert inflict serious harm on the function of several organs. As individuals, we are the products of a constant struggle with our emotions and impulses. Should we seek means to neutralize or manipulate our emotional drive, in order to prevent a perceived harm? Can the end justify the means in this scenario? Furthermore, is it even ethical to minimize or augment emotional feelings via chemicals or "brain washing" methods? Should we set up new standards before new "therapies" become available to us? Consider all the recent uproar regarding stem cell research to grasp how important this debate can be. We aren't there yet, but just imagine the ability to change a person into a fearless being, or to "immunize" against natural emotions such as love, hatred, jealousy, or even loneliness. This is not so ludicrous or far-fetched and may elicit our real attention in the near future.

Drugs are being widely prescribed nowadays, including tranquilizers, mood elevating drugs, and antidepressants. Just imagine what pharmaceutical or physical modalities may become capable of doing. The answers on how to deal with these looming challenges are not readily available. It is, therefore, vital for us to start preparing ourselves from now and to deal with issues before they become too complex to confront, let alone control.

Prevention and management of stress are highly intricate and intensely debated subjects. Resolving the underlying conflict is the main step to recovery. In the majority of cases, this is not as simple as it seems. Other factors entrenched in the psychological makeup of individuals involved may prove to be harder to modify. Examples include difficulties, job related conflicts, financial problems, loneliness, and substance abuse.

Certain general measures can also be of significant help; these include: regular daily exercise, cessation of smoking, avoiding excessive alcohol use, enhancing social activities with family and friends, and a heart-healthy diet. Other activities including meditation, yoga, prayer, music, art appreciation, and reading are frequently prescribed as they seem to provide a positive influence.

YOUR BODY'S OWN SELF DEFENSE

"Too much of a good thing is not necessarily good"! The dictum of "Preservation of species" means that body reactions to any looming danger are intended to help neutralizing the injury and preventing its danger. The variety of hormones released in reaction to acute stress including adrenaline, steroids, angiotensin, and others are meant to keep heart rate and blood pressure high enough to perfuse the brain, the heart, the kidneys, and other vital and particularly vulnerable organs. A combination of rapid "overshoot" and unprepared organs caught off guard can result in unfortunate and unintended damage. A heart muscle overwhelmed with "too much help" faces increased resistance from constricted large arteries, while its own coronary arteries turned spastic may fail to deliver the nutritional supply needed to match the increased demand. This scenario represents unusual reaction to unusual threat. We should remember that in the vast majority of less intense threats, the response, even though of similar nature, is usually more measured and can provide the needed protection without inducing harm.

A SYSTEM OF CHECKS AND BALANCES

If the outside challenge is not overwhelmingly strong, it can be handled by a system of two opposing effects in a manner that helps to restore and later maintains the balance. This process is governed by the so called "Autonomous Nervous System". An adrenergic or sympathetic activity constricts vessels, increases heart rate and blood pressure, while an opposing activity called vagal or parasympathetic does just the opposite. Depending on the circumstances facing the heart and circulation, one of the two will be activated to neutralize the potentially harmful invasion.

Measures Proven To Be Helpful for The Heart

For both prevention and treatment, several lifestyle modifications or interventions are now proven to be effective to stop the drift toward heart failure. Most of these work by minimizing the power of stress reactions or enhancing the calming and modifying influences. Among these measures are:

- Relaxation undoubtedly is beneficial for the heart and circulation. It is believed to work by tempering excessive stimulation and moderating noxious influences. A relaxed or "cool" attitude is admittedly hard to achieve. However, by adhering to special programs of self management, diet, and exercise remarkable levels of self control can be achieved.
- Peaceful environment at work or leisure time, especially when enhanced by calming music. (My personal preference here is Baroque Music).
- Both meditation and yoga exercises imported from the orient have made major headways into western lifestyles. They are believed by many to temper excessive tension, stress, and anxiety.
- Breathing exercises basically utilizing slow and deep breathing, as well as bio-feed back exercises to control chronic stress.
- "Healthy" social relationships within the family, the circle of friends and workplace. Of particular importance here is ridding oneself as much as possible of negative impulses such as jeal-

ousy, hatred, and anger while enhancing positive ones such as altruism, honesty, and realistic levels of expectations.

And Now The Good News
"It is Darkest Before Dawn"

- Amidst the sadness, fear, and frustration, a shining light of hope often leads to the road of recovery. Coming on the heels of a painful experience, heart stunning can only compound the pain. It is good to know that 95% of affected individuals are destined to fully recover within a reasonably short period of time.
- In those who do not, medical treatment for heart failure can provide a great sense of improvement and stability.
- The frequency of this problem in elderly women makes it easier to direct the attention to this group. A high index of suspicion leads to early recognition and treatment and can in turn enhance the already favorable prognosis.
- The small minority of patients in whom the condition deteriorates may often be helped by early interventions that may include heart pacemakers - defibrillators* or heart surgery to replace a damaged valve.
- In predisposed individuals, the practice of relaxation techniques and breathing exercise can result in appreciable preventive benefit.
- There are reasons to believe that high-risk individuals can eventually be scientifically identifiable, and therefore closely observed whenever under emotional distress or any other profoundly stressful experience.
- The ability to manipulate emotions by chemicals or training is still at an early stage. However, even if this becomes a reality, questions will arise as to whether it is ethical or can result in unforeseen complications. We are the products of our emotional experience and dire consequences may result if we recklessly offset our emotional balance.

---

* A small device placed in a patient's chest or abdomen to help control abnormal heart rhythms. The device emits electrical pulses and prompts the heart to beat at a normal rate. Readily available system can convert fatal chaotic rhythm to normal, or synchronize the function of the two ventricles to improve heart output.

WHAT HAVE WE LEARNED?

1. Heart function can be suddenly and severely weakened, "stunned" by a variety of emotional, psychological, social, and neurogenic conditions.

2. Most frequently encountered causes include the loss of loved ones, surprising mass disasters, shocking news, and acute stressful situations.

3. The resulting "Broken Heart" is, in most cases, self-limited with recovery of heart function expected within 1-2 weeks. Nevertheless, protracted weakness and occasional death have been reported in a small percentage of patients.

4. The condition occurs predominantly in women after menopause.

5. A host of chemicals including adrenaline, other catecholamines, and neurohormonal transmitters are almost certainly the major mediators of heart stunning.

6. Cocaine and amphetamine abuse should always be considered in unexplained heart attacks and heart failure, especially in young people.

7. Depression and chronic stress also predispose to heart weakness and spasm of coronary arteries that supply nutritional need to the heart muscle. Post Traumatic Stress Disorder (PTSD) can, in addition, contribute to premature hardening of heart arteries (atherosclerosis)

8. Life-style modifications, relaxation techniques, and psychosocial management may all be helpful in the prevention and treatment of this syndrome. Certain medications and interventions are frequently effective in speeding the recovery and preventing sudden or progressive worsening.

Sources:

1. Akashi YJ Nakazawa K, et al. The clinical features of Takotsubo cardiomyopathy. QJM 2003;96:563
2. Allegra JR, Mostashari F, et al. Cardiac events in New Jersey after the September 11, 2001, terrorist attack. *J Urban Health* 2005;82:358
3. Bashour TT, Myler RK, et al. Current concepts in unstable myocardial ischemia. Am Heart J 1988;115:850
4. Bashour T, Cheng TO. Profound repolarization abnormality and cardiomyopathy in pheochromocytoma. Chest 1976;70:397
5. Bashour T, Fandul H, et al. Electrocardiographic findings in alcoholic cardiomyopathy, a study of 65 patients. Chest 1975;68:24
6. Bashour T, hakim 0, et al. severe coronary spasm with sinus node dysfunction. Archives of Internal Medicine 1982;142:1719
7. Bashour T, hakim 0, et al. Vasospastic angina in middle-aged women. A psychosomatic disorder? American Heart Journal 1983;106:609
8. Bashour T, Kabbani S, et al. sinus node dysfunction and cardiac failure during vasospastic angina. American Heart Journal 1984;108:1056
9. Bashour T, Kabbani S, et al. transient Q waves and cardiac failure during ischemia. Electrical and mechanical "stunning" of the heart. American Heart Journal 1983;106:780
10. Bashour T. Cardiac rhythm disorders associated with coronary spasm, Clinical Cardiology 1984;7:510
11. Bashour T, Hanna E, et al. Myocardial revascularization with internal mammary artery bypass. An emerging treatment of choice. American Heart Journal 1986;111:143
12. Bashour T. Myocardial life, hibernation and death (editorial). American Heart Journal 1986;112:427
13. Bashour T, Hanna E, et al. Open heart surgery in patients above the age of eighty. Clinical Cardiology 1990;13:26793
14. Bashour T, Morelli R, et al. Acute coronary thrombosis following head trauma in a young man. American Heart Journal 1990;119:676
15. Bashour T, Mason D, et al. Cardiomyopathies: current diagnosis and treatment. Primary Cardiology 1989;15:29

16. Bashour T. Vasotonic myocardial ischemia (review). American Heart Journal 1991;122:1701

17. Bashour T. Vasotonic acute myocardial infarction: Experience with eight cases. Int. J. Angiology 1993;2:82

18. Bashour T. Acute myocardial infarction resulting from amphetamine abuse. A Spasm-Thrombus interplay? American Heart Journal 1994;128:1237

19. Brandspiegel HZ, Marinchak RA, et al. A broken Heart. Circulation 1998;98:1349

20. Braunwald E, Kloner RA. The stunned myocardium: prolonged, post ischemic ventricular dysfunction. Circulation. 1982;66: 1146

21. Cheng TO, Bashour T, et al: Myocardial infarction in the absence of coronary arteriosclerosis. Result of coronary spasm? American Journal of Cardiology 1972;30:680

22. Cheng TO, Bashour T, et al. Variant angina of Prinzmetal with normal coronary arteriograms. A variant of the variant. Circulation 1973;47:475

23. Culic V, Eterovic D, et al. Meta-analysis of possible external triggers of acute myocardial infarction. Int J Cardiol 2005;99:1

24. Culic V, Miric D, et al. Different circumstances timing, and symptom presentation at onset of Q waves versus non-Q wave acute myocardial infarction. Am J Cardiol 2002;89:456

25. Desmet WI, Adriaenssens BF, et al. Apical ballooning of the left ventricle: first series in white patients. Heart 2003;89:1027

26. Dionsdale JE. Psychological Stress and Cardiovascular Disease. J. AM. Coll. Cardiology 2008; 51; 13:1237

27. Donohue D, Movahed MR. Clinical characteristics, demographics and prognosis of transient left ventricular apical ballooning syndrome. *Heart Fail Rev* 2005;10:311

28. Dote K, Sato H, et al. Myocardial stunning due to simultaneous multivessel coronary spasms: a review of 5 cases (in Japanese).*J Cardiol.* 1991;21(2):203

29. Engle GL. Sudden and rapid death during psychological stress: folklore or folk wisdom. *Ann Intern Med.* 1971;74:771

30. Fagring AJ; Kjellgren K, et al: Depression, anxiety, stress, social interaction, and related quality of life in men and women with unexplained chest pain. Bio Med Central 2008; May 19

31. Ganz W. Coronary spasm in myocardial infarction: fact or fiction? Circulation 1981;63:487

32. Gianni M, Dentali F, et al. Apical ballooning syndrome or Takotsubo cardiomyopathy: a systematic review. *Eur Heart J2006;27:1523*

33. Heupler FJ Jr. Syndrome of symptomatic coronary arterial spasm with nearly normal coronary arteriograms. *Am J Cardiol* 1980;45:873

34. Heupler FA, Proudfit WA, et al. Ergonovine maleate provocative test for coronary arterial spasm. Am J Cardiol 1978;41:631

35. Kurisu S, Sato H, et al. Tako-tsubo like left ventricular dysfunction with ST segment elevation: a novel cardiac syndrome mimicking acute myocardial infarction. Am Heart J 2002;143:448

36. Lam YTT, Chesebro JH, et al. Is vasospasm related to platelet deposition? Relationship in a porcine preparation or arterial injury in vivo. Circulation 1987;78:243

37. Latham PM. Collected works. Vol I. London: New Sydenham Society, 1876:445

38. Lee VII, Connolly HM, et al. Tako-tsubo cardiomyopathy in aneurismal subarachnoid hemorrhage: an underappreciated ventricular dysfunction. J Neurosurg 2006;105:264

39. Leor J. Kloner RA. The Northridge earthquake as a trigger for acute myocardial infarction. *Am J Cardiol.* 1996;77:1230

40. Leor J, Poole WK, et al. Sudden cardiac death triggered by an earthquake. *N Engl J mMed.* 1996;334:413

41. Maseri A, Mimmo R, et al. A Coronary artery spasm as a cause of acute myocardial ischemia in man. Chest 1975;68:625

42. Maseri A, L'Abbate A, et al. Coronary vasospasm in angina pectoris. Lancet 1977;1:713

43. Maseri A. Pathogenetic mechanism of angina pectoris: expanding views. *Br Heart J*1980;43:648

44. Maseri A, Severi S, et al. "Variant" angina: one aspect of a continuous spectrum of vasospastic myocardial ischemia. Pathogenetic mechanism, estimated incidence and clinical coronary arteriographic findings In 138 patients. *Am J Cordial* 1978;42:1019

45. Maseri A, Chierchia S, et al. Pathophysiology of coronary occlusion in acute myocardial infarction. Circulation 1986;73:233

46. McCord J,, Jneid H, et al. Management of Cocaine—associated chest pain and myocardial infarction. Circulation 117 & 1897, 2008

47. Meisel SR, Kutz I, et al. Effect of Iraqi missile war on incidence of acute myocardial infarction and sudden death in Israeli civilians. *Lancet* 1991;338:660

48. Mori H, Ishikawa S, et al. Increased Responsiveness of left ventricular apical myocardium to adrenergic stimuli. *Cardiovasc Res.* 1993;27:192

49. Nanda AS, Feldman A, et al. Acute reversal of pheochromocytoma-induced catecholamine cardiomyopathy. *Clin Cardiol 1995;* 18:421

50. O'Connor M, Allen J, et al. Autonomic and emotion regulation in bereavement and depression. *J Psychosom Res.* 2002;52:183

51. Osier W. Lumleian lecture on angina pectoris. Lecture I. Lancet 1910;697

52. Otomo S, Sugita M, et al. Two cases of transient left ventricular apical ballooning syndrome associated with subarachnoid hemorrhage. Anesthesia & Analgesia. 103, 3:583, 2006

53. Palmer RMJ, Ferrige AG, et al. Nitric oxide release accounts for the biological activity of endothelium-derived relaxing factor. Nature 1987;327:524

54. *Parodi G, Acute Emotional stress and cardiac arrhythmia. JAMA.* 2007;298 (3):324

55. Pavin D, Le Breton H, et al. Human stress cardiomyopathy mimicking acute myocardial syndrome. Heart 1997;78:509

56. Prinzmetal M, Ekemecki A, et al. Variant form of angina pectoris: previously underlineated syndrome. JAMA 1960;174:791

57. Sharkey SW, Lesser JR, et al. Acute and reversible cardiomyopathy provoked by stress in women from the United States. *Circulation* 2005; 111:472

58. Sharkey SW, Windenberg Dc, et al. Natural history and expansive clinical profile of stress cardiomyopathy. *Journal of the Amer. Coll. Of Cardiology 2010 5534:333-341.*

59. Tofler GH, Muller JE. Triggering of acute cardiovascular disease and potential preventive strategies. Circulation 2006; 114:1863

60. Torpy, Janet, et al. Chronic stress and the heart. JAMA. 2007; 298 (14): 1722

61. Tsuchihashi K, Ueshima K, et al. Transient left ventricular apical ballooning without coronary artery stenosis: a novel

heart syndrome mimicking acute myocardial infarction. J Am Coll Cardiol 2001;38;11

62. Valente AM, Bashore TM. Unusual cardiomyopathies; ventricular noncompaction and tokotsubo cardiomyopathy. *Rev Cardiovasc Med* 2006;7:111

63. Villareal RP, Achari A, et al. Anteroapical stunning and left ventricular outflow tract obstruction. Mayo Clin Proc 2001;76:79

64. Watanabe H, Kodama M, et al. earthquakes and Takotsubo cardiomyopathy. JAMA *2005;294:2169*

65. Witte DR, Bois MI, et al. Cardiovascular mortality in Dutch men during 1996 European football championship: longitudinal population study. *BMJ* 2000;321:1552

66. Wittstein IS, Thiemann DR, et al. Neurohumoral features of myocardial stunning due to sudden emotional stress. *N Engl J Med* 2005;352:539

67. Yamanaka O, Yasumasa F, et al. "Myocardial stunning" like phenomenon during a crisis of pheochromocytoma. Jpn Circ J 1994;58:737

68. Yasue H, Touyama M, et al. Prinzmetal's variant form of angina as a manifestation of alpha-adrenergic receptor mediated coronary artery spasm: documentation by coronary arteriography. *Am Heart J.1976;* 91:148

69. Young M, Benjamin B, et al. the mortality of widowers. *Lancet* 1963;2:454

70. Zlegelstein RC. Acute emotional stress and cardiac arrhythmias. JAMA. 2007; 298 (3): 324

Figures:

FIG. 1

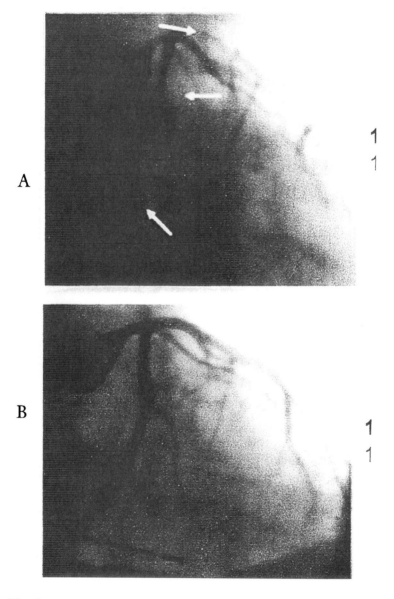

A

B

Fig. 1
A. Extensive Coronary Artery Spasm
B. Normalization after nitroglycerine injection

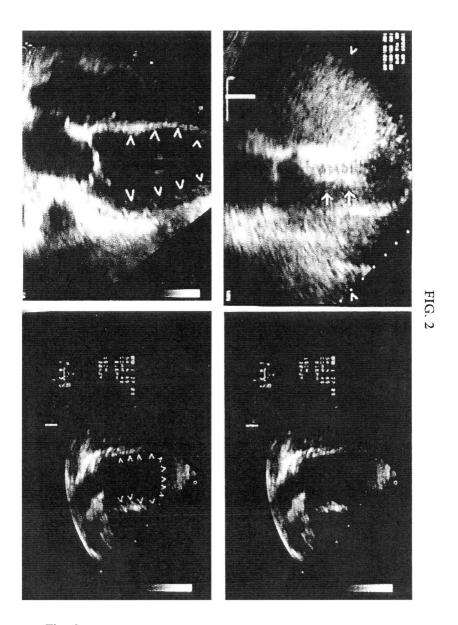

FIG. 2

Fig. 2

Four Echo Cardiogram images of enlarged and weakened hearts after emotional shock.

FIG. 3

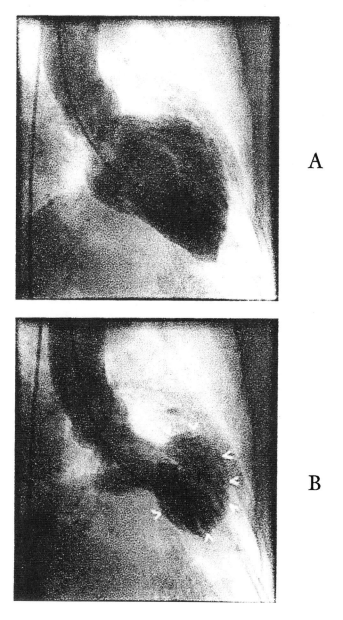

Fig 3
A. Angiographic image of enlarged heart after emotional shock.
B. During contraction the apex of the heart does not move "arrow heads" (Tako-tsubo syndrome).